Technical Bulletin
VoL V No. 2

HANDBOOK ON PHILIPPINE MEDICINAL PLANTS
Volume III

Ludivina S. de Padua
Gregorio C. Lugod
Juan V. Pancho

Published by the Documentation and Information Section
Office of the Director of Research
University of the Philippines at Los Baños

College of Arts and Sciences
University of the Philippines at Los Baños
College, Laguna
1st Printing, February 1981
2nd Printing, November 1982

The authors wish to express their gratitude for the assistance of the following: Mrs. M. B. Quimzon, Mrs. V. E. Concio, Miss E. C. Velasco, Miss C. G. Lantican and Mr. Felix Aquino.

Acknowledgements are also due Dr. E. D. Reyes, Director of Research, Mrs. Z. Z. Cabrera for the book and cover design, and the staff of the Documentation and Information Section of the Office of the Director of Research, UPLB.

The authors also acknowledge the financial assistance extended by the National Science Development Board (NSDB) for the printing of the book.

Part of this undertaking was funded by the UPLB Basic Research Project 75-9.

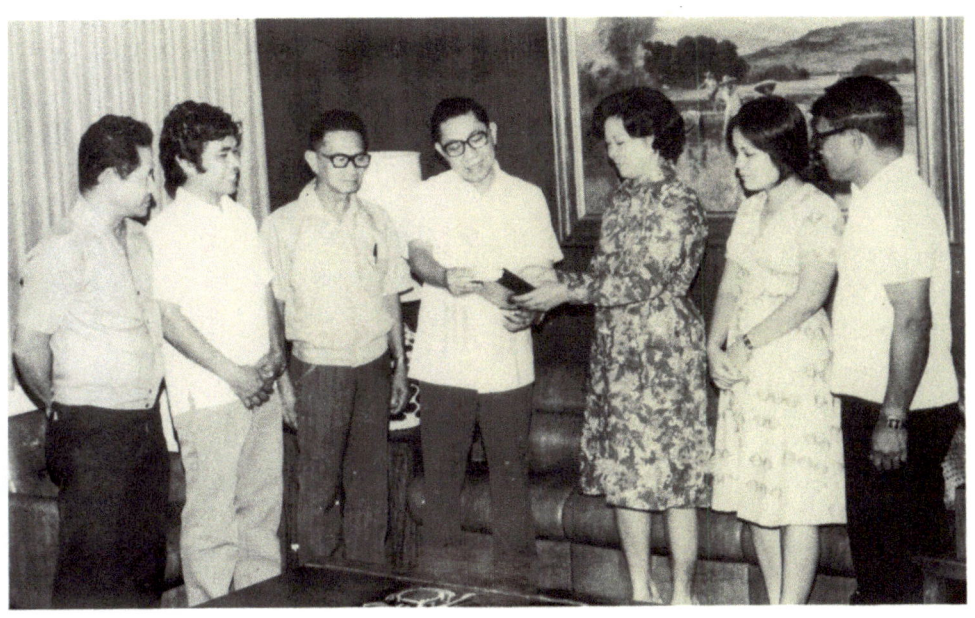

FIRST VOLUME: Prof Ludivina S. de Padua presents Volume I of Handbook on Philippine Medicinal Plants to the late UPLB Chancellor Abelardo G. Samonte, November 23, 1977. L to r: Dr. E. D. Reyes, Director of Research, Dr. B. T. Mercado, Chairman, Botany Dept., Prof. G. C. Lugod, co-author, Chancellor Samonte, Prof. De Padua, Mrs. Z. Z. Cabrera, editor and cover designer, representing the Documentation and Information Section, publisher of the handbook, and Prof. J. V. Pancho, co-author.

Contents

31	*Orthosiphon aristatus* (*Balbas-pusa*)	42	*Cardiospermum halicacabum* (*Parol-parolan*)
32	*Adenanthera pavonina* (*Saga*)	43	*Manilkara zapota* (*Chico*)
33	*Aloe barbadensis* (*Sabila*)	44	*Nicotiana tabacum* (*Tabaco*)
34	*Strychnos nux-vomica* (*Strychnine plant*)	45	*Solanum melongena* (*Talong*)
35	*Donax cannaeformis* (*Bamban*)	46	*Solanum nigrum* (*Lubi-lubi*)
36	*Ficus elastica* (*Balete*)	47	*Duranta repens* (*Golden dew drop*)
37	*Piper nigrum* (*Paminta*)	48	*Lantana camara* (*Kantutay*)
38	*Pittosporum pentandrum* (*Mamalis*)	49	*Costus speciosus* (*Spiral ginger*)
39	*Plantago major* (*Lanting*)	50	*Curcuma zedoaria* (*Barak*)
40	*Gardenia jasminoides* (*Rosal*)	51	*Kaempferia galanga* (*Duso*)
41	*Triphasia trifolia* (*Limoncito*)		

Introduction

EVIDENCE of the significance being increasingly attached to medicinal plants is the successful introduction in recent years of various drugs of natural origin, as well as the continuing effort of the pharmaceutical industry in the search for natural sources of new drugs from different parts of the world. Some drug manufacturers are sending their own botanical explorers to distant lands, and research agencies are laboring to discover new materials that would be of importance in the solution of many critical health problems. Until recently, both scientific and practical information on medicinal plants have often been inadequate or entirely lacking.

Much emphasis has been placed on the production and utilization of plants and the products derived from them in meeting world food problems. Equal concern and importance should be given to human health and the proper utilization of medicinal plants in the efforts towards the improvement of health conditions. Unfortunately, this aspect of man's use of plants has not received much attention, either in terms of research priority or publicity as has the food and feed aspect. In the last decade however, Filipino scientists, mainly through individual efforts and sheer dedication, have begun to prove the scientific basis for the use of these plants in medicine.

Preparation of the Handbook on Philippine Medicinal Plants was undertaken with the main objective of disseminating information and the creation of an awareness of the importance of our medicinal plants as well as their proper utilization. Volume 1 was printed in September 1977, and volume 2 in November 1978. Like the first two volumes, this book is a collection of fifty more medicinal plants, with information such as scientific name, common names, the family to which the plant belongs, description, ecological distribution, reported medicinal value, manner of administration, and histochemical findings for each plant. Color reproductions of photographs of the plants are included in this volume.

Plants are a particularly interesting source of important substances since they provide chemicals with structures not likely to be synthesized in the laboratory. These plant products may be acting synergistically or antagonistically in producing the activity necessary in the treatment of diseases. Histochemical tests were conducted on these plants and the findings are recorded in the text as: 1 = detectable, 2 = abundant, 3 = very abundant, in the plant parts where the particular constituent was found present.

One other objective of publishing this book is conservation. Many people still do not recognize these medicinal plants that are all around us. These plants are oftentimes in danger of being destroyed and completely eradicated. Our concern about conservation of our natural resources extends beyond aesthetics and environmental protection. It is imperative that an adequate and continuous supply of medicinal plants is assured; it is therefore necessary to be very conservation-conscious.

Plants have played an important role in traditional medicine from the earliest times. Medicinal plants, and the arbularyo (herbolario) are part of our cultural heritage. Plant products have been used in the treatment of diseases for many years and could be considered historically to be the first drugs. The goal of traditional medicine and that of modern medicine are the same — the improvement of man's health. Perhaps in the near future, plants will play an even greater role than their present highly significant one.

L.S. de Padua

1

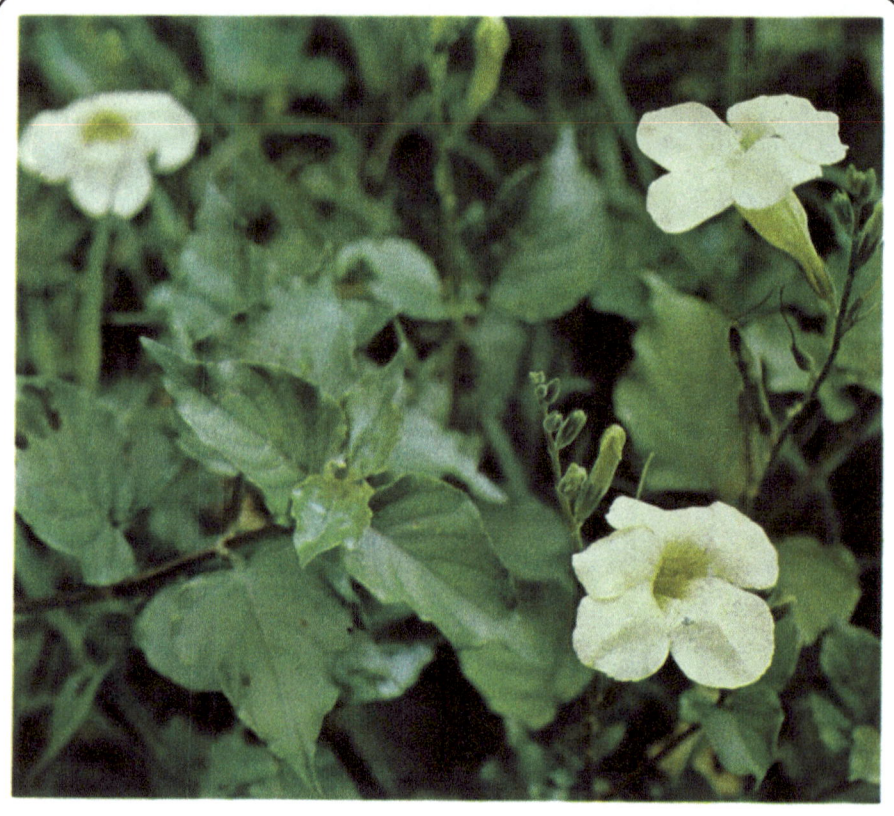

ACANTHACEAE
Asystasia gangetica (L.) T. Anders.
Asistasia, zamboangenita (in most dialects)

Procumbent herb, growing up to 1 m or more in height. The leaves are ovate, 2.5 to 3 cm wide, the tip is pointed and the base rounded or suddenly narrowed. The flowers are borne in lax racemes 5 to 12 cm. in length. The sepals are linear-lanceolate, about 5 mm long and hairy on the back. Corolla is hairy and 2.5 to 3 cm long with an inflated yellow tube, the limb is pink or pale purple, usually dull or lucid, and sometimes yellow altogether. The capsule is cylindric, compressed, about 2.5 cm long and hairy. The seeds are smooth, much compressed, ovoid, angular, wrinkled and less than 5 mm in diameter.

Widely distributed in the Philippines.

Leaf is an antidote for snake bite. Juice is vermifuge, for rheumatism and swelling. Decoction is an intestinal astringent and used as enema for pregnant women to lighten childbirth.

Tannin in stem = 1; saponin, leaves and stem = 1-2; calcium oxalate, stem = 2.

2

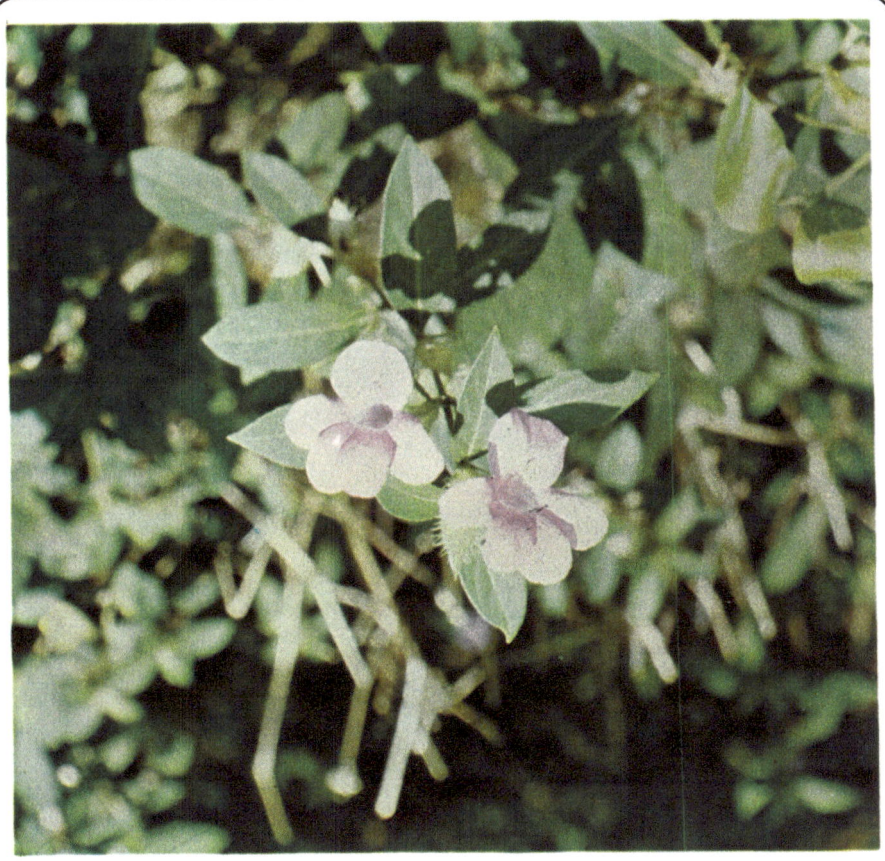

ACANTHACEAE
Barleria cristata L.
Violeta (Sp.); *Kolintang, violeta* (Tag.).

An erect, much-branched shrub 1 to 3 m high, the branches sparingly pubescent. Leaves oblong to elliptic, acute, 4 to 10 cm long, somewhat pubescent beneath. Flowers in the upper axils and terminal, solitary or in pairs, the bracteoles linear. Outer two sepals green ovate-lanceolate, nearly 2 cm long, persistent, laciniate-toothed. Corolla 6 to 7 cm long, the tube slender, winged above, the limb 4 to 5 cm in diameter, violet or nearly white, or streaked with violet and white.

Commonly cultivated, especially as a hedge plant. A native of India, now cultivated in many tropical countries.

The roots and leaves are used to reduce swellings. Infusion of roots and leaves is given for coughs. Seeds are used as an antidote for snake-bite.

Calcium oxalate in stem = 2; fats in stem = 1-2; pectic substances in leaf and stem = 1; formic acid in stem = 1.

3

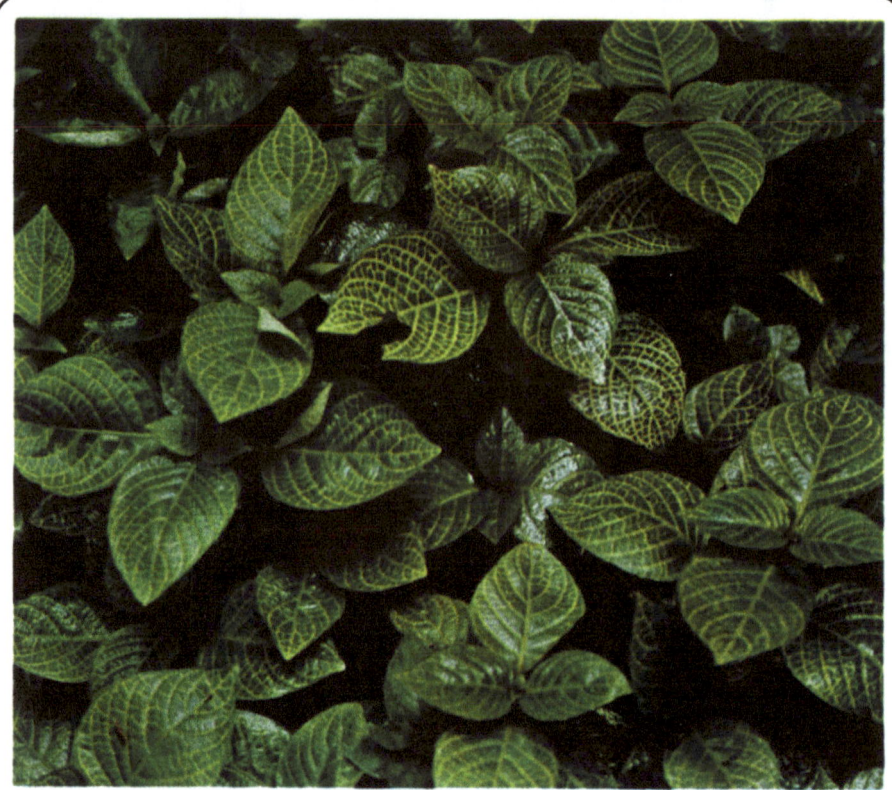

ACANTHACEAE
Blechum pyramidatum (Lam.) Urban (= *B. brownei* Juss.)
Dayang, sapin-sapin (Tag.); *bamburia, tari-tari, karimbusuk, kopis-kopis* (Ilk.).

An erect ascending herb, the stems often prostrate and rooting below, 20 to 50 cm high, sparingly hairy or nearly glabrous. Leaves thin, ovate 5 to 10 cm long, entire or nearly so, acute, base decurrent, acuminate. Inflorescence terminal, spike-like, the flowers mostly in pairs, each pair subtended by a leaf-like, ovate, persistent, 1 to 1.5 cm long bract and two smaller bracteoles. Flowers small, white. Calyx 4 to 5 mm long, hairy, five-lobed, the lobes linear. Corolla white, tubular, hairy, slightly curved, about 1.3 cm long, slightly exerted from the bracts. Capsule ovoid, acuminate, somewhat compressed about 6 mm long.

Found in waste places, roadsides, etc., widely distributed in the Philippines.

Entire plant in decoction is used as an antiblenorrhagic. Pounded leaves are employed as vulnerary.

Tannin in leaves = 2, stem   saponin in leaves   = 1, stem = 1-2; amylodextrin in stem = 1; phytosterol in leaves = 1, stem = 2.

4

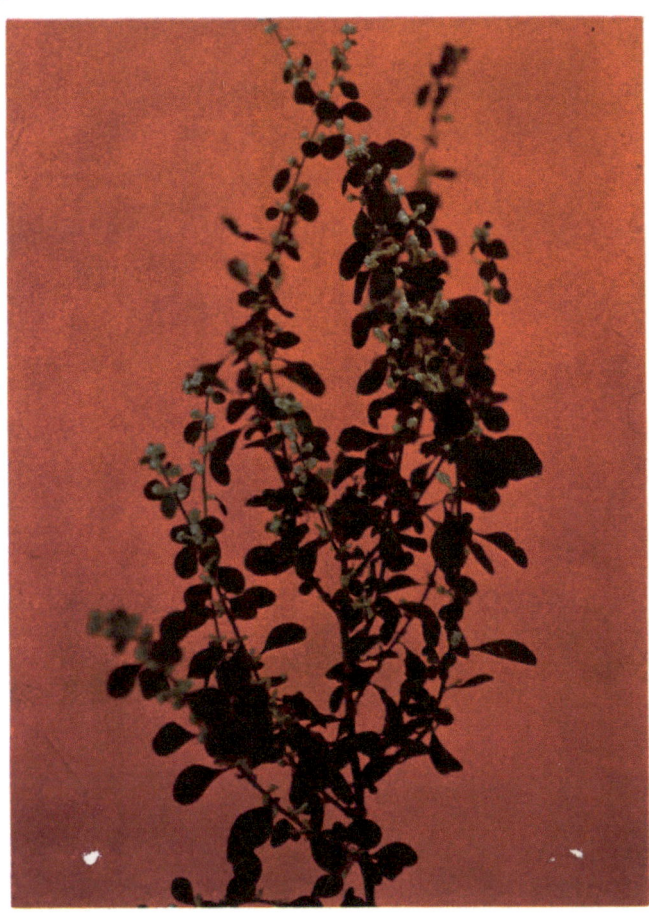

AMARANTHACEAE
Aerva lanata (L.) Juss.
Tabang-ahas; apug-apugan, pamaynap (Tag.); *karlatan* (Ilk.).

An ascending or prostrate, densely grayish-pubescent herb, the stems 0.2 to 0.8 m in length, simple or branched. Leaves alternate, petioled, elliptic to orbicular or obovate, obtuse, 1 to 3.5 cm long. Spikes numerous, white, axillary, solitary or crowded in the axils, densely flowered, 1 cm long or less, the flowers green and white, 2 mm in diameter.

Found in open dry lands, common throughout the Philippines at low altitudes.

Plant decoction is for bladder affections, anthelmintic, vermifuge for children, for cough.

Saponin in leaves and stem = 2; calcium oxalate, stem = 1, leaves = 2; pectic substances, leaves = 1.

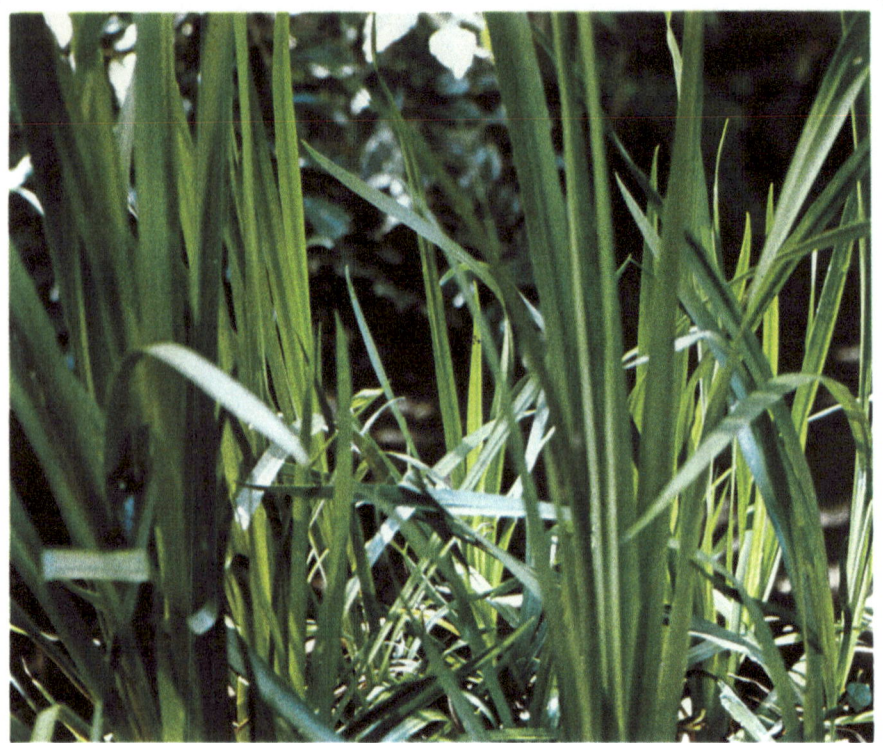

ARACEAE
Acorus calamus L.
Lubigan (Tag., Bis.); *bueng* (Pamp.); *acoro* (Sp.); *daraw, dalaw* (Ilk.);
dengaw (Bon.); Sweet flag (Engl.).

Aromatic, perennial herb with creeping, branching, and stout rootstock, whitish to yellowish inside the rhizome. Leaves linear, flat, smooth, acuminate, 25 to 60 cm long, 1 to 1.5 cm. wide. Peduncle compressed. Spathe green, much-elongated, similar in shape to the leaves. Spadix 3-5 cm long, 1 cm or less in diameter. Sepals 6, stamens 6, rarely flowering in the Philippines. Fruit berries turbinate, prismatic with pyramidal tops. Underground rhizome slender and crooked.

Occasionally cultivated.

The rootstock is used as a diarrhea remedy; stomachic, tonic, aphrodisiac and carminative. Decoction of the rhizome is emetic, antispasmodic, and has been used as a remedy for asthma, chronic dysentery and as a tonic; is a stimulant, expectorant and anti-dyspeptic. Crushed rhizome is applied as an embrocation in rheumatism; powdered and mixed with oil, it is used externally for fungal skin diseases and scabies. Powdered root is insecticidal.

Alkaloid in rhizome = 1-2; saponin in rhizome = 1-2; sulfur, rhizome = 1-2; fats in leaves = 1; glycosides in rhizome = 1.

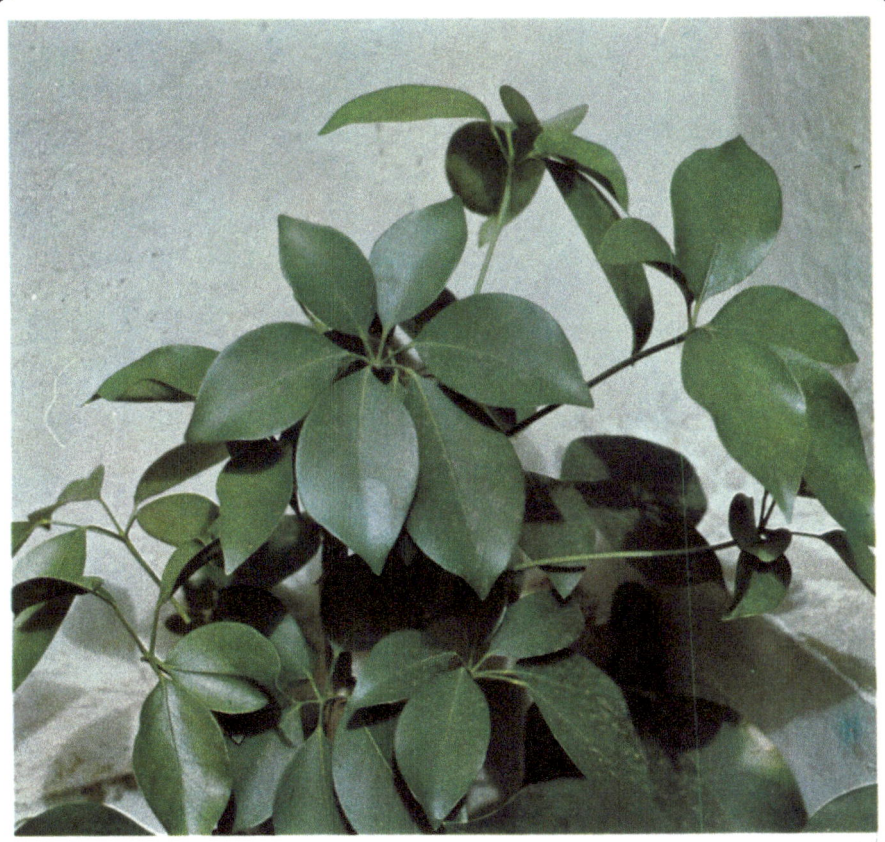

ARALIACEAE

Schefflera odorata (Blanco) Merr. & Rolfe.

Arasagot (Ilk.); *galamay-amo, lima-lima*(Tag.); *kalakang* (Bag.); *karangkang, kayangkang, kokontimbalun* (Yak.); *palan* (Sul.); *panayang* (Tagb.); *tagima* (Bis., Yak.); *tagilima, tuglima* (Bis.); *tarangkang* (S.L. Bis.); *tughik* (Iv.).

A glabrous vine, reaching a height of 2 to 6 m or more. Petioles longer than the leaflets. Leaflets 5 to 6, smooth and shining, coriaceous, elliptic to broadly ovate, obtuse or very shortly acuminate, 6 to 12 cm long. Panicles terminal, lax 10 to 20 cm long. Flowers greenish, 2 to 3 mm in diameter. Fruits globose and fleshy when fresh, 4 to 5 mm long, prominently and sharply six-angled when dry.

Widely distributed in the Philippines.

Bark decoction is a remedy for cough. Decoction of leaves antiscorbutic. Resin is employed as vulnerary.

Tannin, leaves and stem = 1; saponin in leaves = 1, stem = 1-2; calcium oxalate in leaves = 1, stem = 1-2; fats, leaves = 1, stem = 1-2.

7

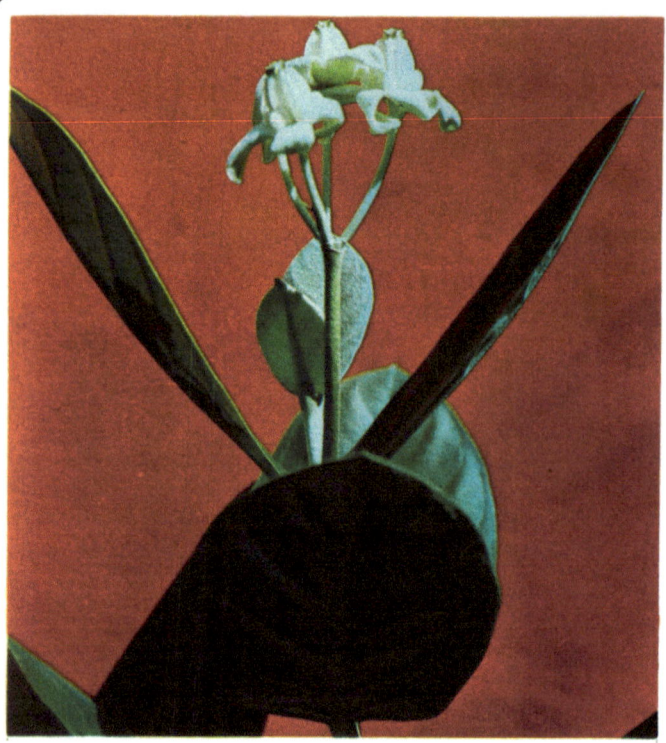

ASCLEPIADACEAE
Calotropis gigantea (Willd.) Dryand. ex W.T. Ait.
Kapal-kapal (Tag.); gigantic shallow-wort, mudar (Engl.).

Medium-sized shrub, growing from 2 to 3 m in height. The young parts are covered with appressed white hairs. Bark pale. The leaves cottony beneath, pointed at the tip and heart-shaped at the base. Flowers have a faint odor, downy on the outside, arranged in axillary or sub-terminal, simple or compound inflorescences. Corolla 1.5 to 2.5 cm across, usually white, sometimes dull-purple or purplish-lilac. Lobes ovate-lanceolate, spreading. Fruit 7.5 to 10 cm long, recurved. Seeds ovate, 5 to 6 mm long, furnished with a bright silky-white coma.

Cultivated in Manila and other large towns in the Philippines. Introduced from tropical Asia, and is now pantropic in cultivation.

The leaves, warmed and moistened with oil are applied as a dry fomentation for abdominal pains and also make a good rubefacient. The juice of young buds is a remedy for earache. The powdered bark is emetic. The root, made into an ointment is used in the treatment of old ulcers and other skin diseases.

Tannin in leaves = 1; stem = 1-2; saponin in leaves and stem = 1; calcium oxalate in leaves = 1, stem = 2.

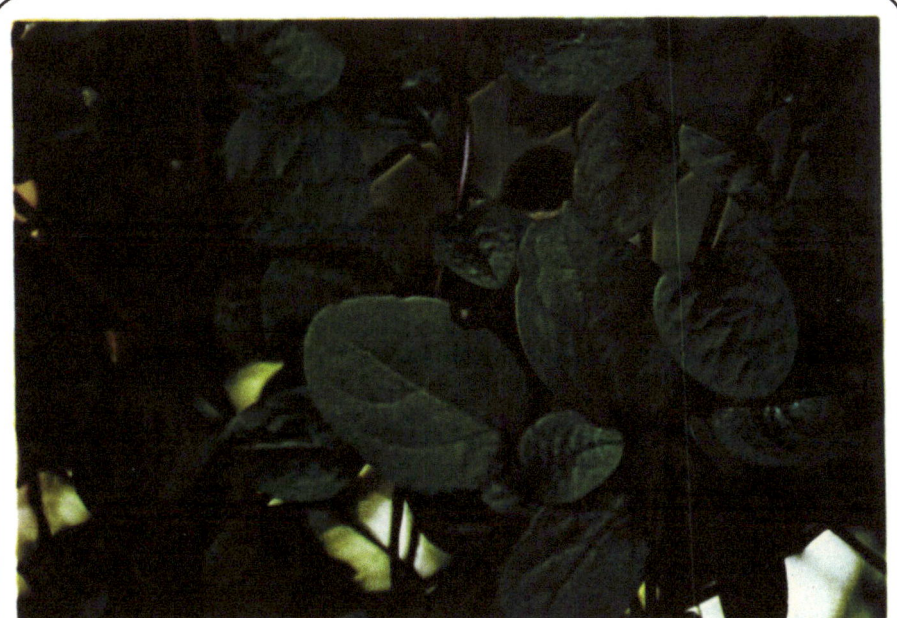

BASELLACEAE
Basella alba L.
Alugbati, libato, grana (Tag.); *ilaibakir* (Ilk.); *alugbati* (Bis.);
arogbati (Bik.); *dundula* (Sul.); Malabar nightshade, vine spinach (Engl.)

This is a succulent, branched, smooth, twining, herbaceous vine, reaching a length of several meters. The stems are green or purplish. The leaves are somewhat fleshy, ovate or heart-shaped, 5 to 12 cm in length, stalked, tapering to a pointed tip, and cordate at the base. The spikes are axillary, solitary, and 5 to 20 cm in length. The flowers are pink, and about 4 mm long. The fruit is fleshy, stalkless, ovoid or nearly spherical, 5 to 6 mm in length, and purple when mature.

Found in settled areas in hedges, used as vegetable throughout the Philippines.

Roots are employed as rubefacient and poultice to reduce local swellings. Leaves are used for boils and ulcers; as mild laxative for pregnant women.

Calcium oxalate in leaves = 2, stem = 1; starch in leaves = 1, stem = 2; saponin in leaves = 1.

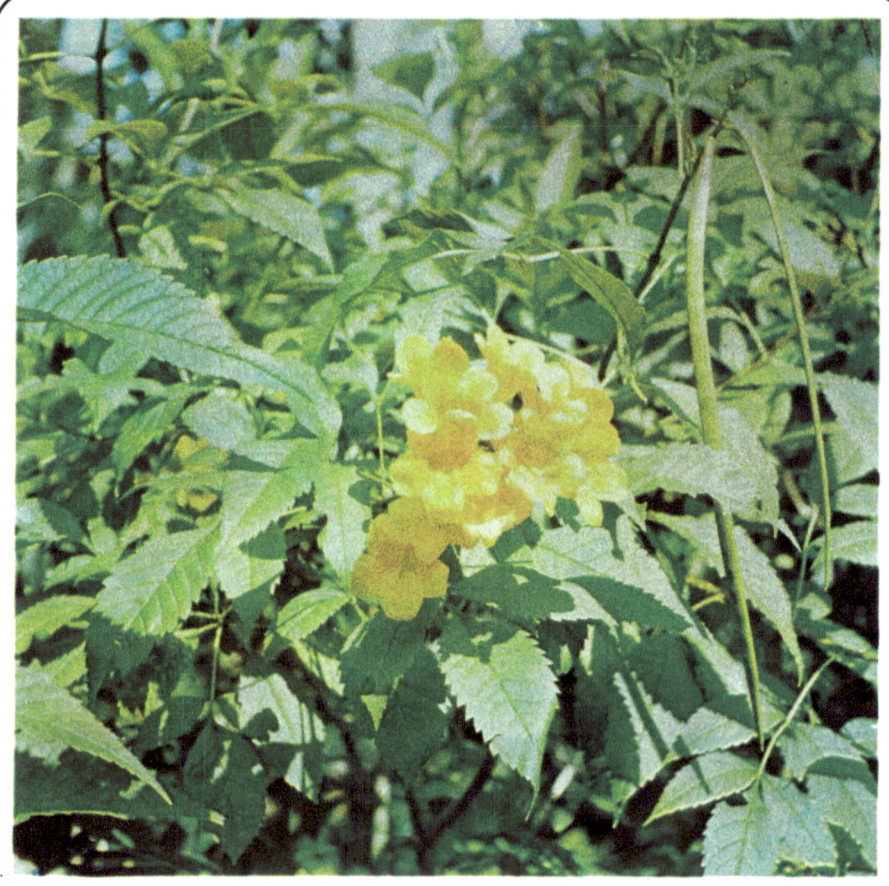

BIGNONIACEAE
Tecoma stans (.) H.B.K.
Yellow bell, yellow elder (Engl.).

An erect, branched, sparingly pubescent or nearly glabrous shrub, 2 to 4 m high. Leaves opposite, odd-pinnate, up to 20 cm in length, leaflets five or seven, lanceolate to oblong-lanceolate, 6 to 13 cm long, long and slenderly acuminate, base acute or acuminate, margins sharply serrate. Panicles terminal. Flowers racemosely arranged on the few branches. Calyx green, 5 mm long, five-toothed. Corolla yellow, 4 to 4.5 cm long, tube inflated upward. Capsules linear, about 15 cm long, 8 mm wide, acuminate, compressed.

Occasionally cultivated for ornamental purposes in some parts of the Philippines. A native of tropical America.

The roots are reported to be a powerful diuretic and tonic. Vermifuge properties are ascribed to the plant. A decoction of the flowers and bark is administered for pains in the stomach; and is said to be good for diabetes.

Tannin in stem = 1-2; amygdalin, stem = 1; calcium oxalate in stem = 1.2.

10

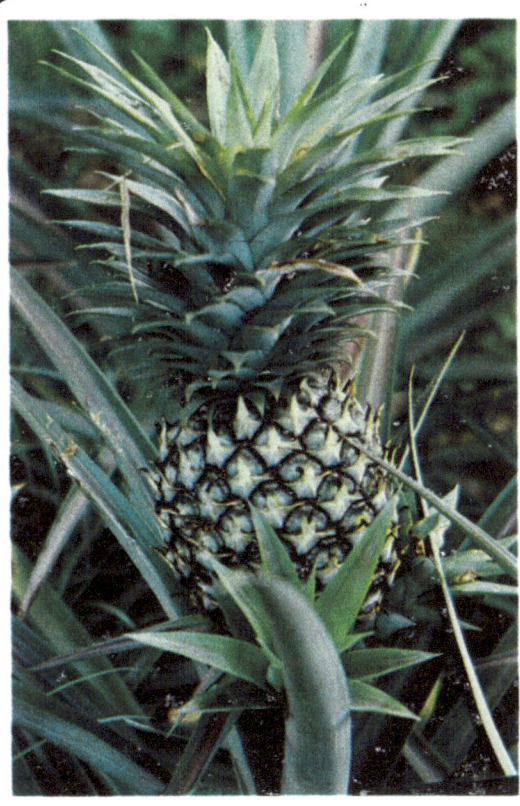

BROMELIACEAE
Ananas comosus (L.) Merr.
Pinya (most dialects); pineapple (Engl.).

It has numerous strong, sword-shaped leaves with pair-toothed edges in rosette, topped by a dense head of flowers. The leaves about 70 to 80 are quite
rigid and concave on the upper side. The small stalkless flowers, which are
reddish-purple, are thickly crowded on an axis and mature into the fleshy
elongated body that is known as the "pineapple." The compound inflorescence may contain 100 to 200 flowers aligned in three spiral rows.
Flowering occurs from the base to the apex. The perfect flowers has parts in
3's. It is subtended by a fleshy thickened bract tapering into a papery tip.
The 3 sepals project beyond the calyx with two fleshy scales at the base. The
inferior ovary has a fleshy style ending into three pale violet stigmas.

Commonly cultivated throughout the Philippines.

Leaf juice is regarded as anthelmintic, purgative, and anti-inflammatory.
The unripe fruit is considered to be diuretic, anthelmintic, expectorant and
abortifacient, and is also credited with emmenagogue properties. Bruised
plant is applied to burns, itches and boils.

Calcium oxalate in leaves = 1-2; pectic substances in leaves = 1.

11

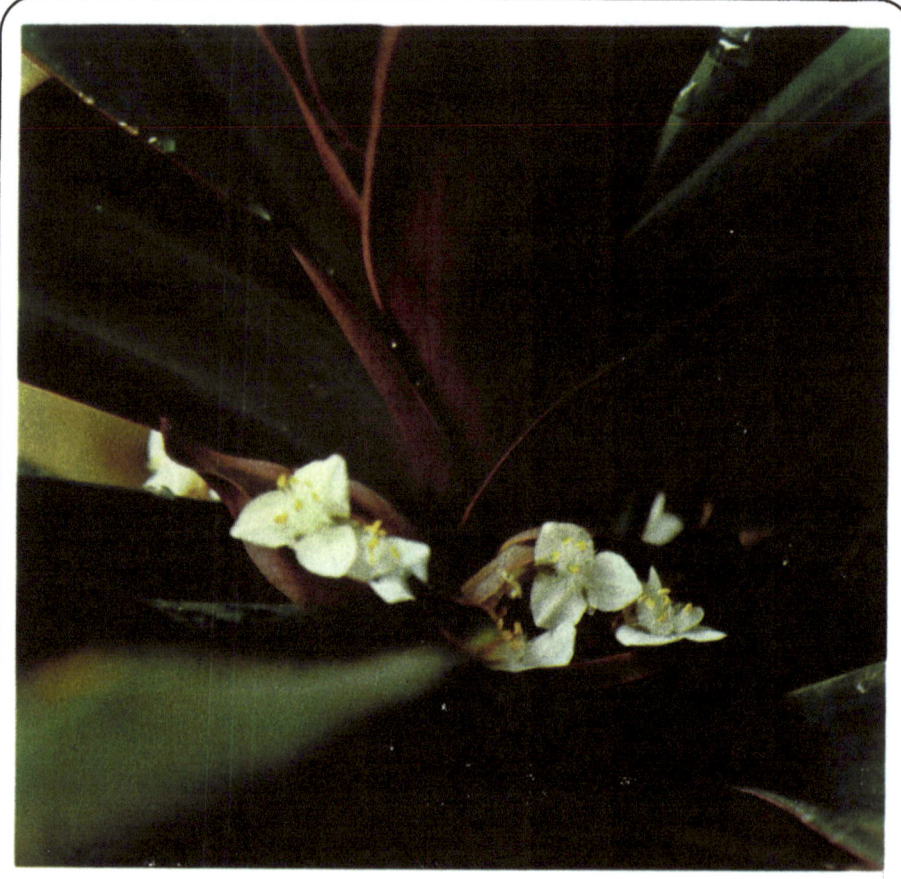

COMMELINACEAE
Rhoeo spathacea (Swartz) W.T. Stearn [= *R. discolor* (L'Herit.) Hance].
Bangka-bangkaan (Tag.); boat lily (Engl.).

A stout, perennial, herbaceous, somewhat fleshy plant, 0.5 m in height or less, the stem thick and unbranched. Leaves lanceolate, acuminate, 40 to 60 cm long, 4 to 6 cm wide, fleshy, the upper surface dark green, the lower purple. Flowers numerous in each inflorescence, fascicled, white, about 1 cm in diameter. Inflorescence axillary, short, peduncled, the flowers surrounded by two large, imbricate, laterally compressed, distichous 3 to 4 cm long, purplish bracts.

Planted for ornamental purposes throughout the Philippines.

Decoction of flowers and leaves is a remedy for colds, whooping cough, nosebleed, bacillary dysentery and blood in stool.

Calcium oxalate in leaves and stem = 1, fatty substances in leaves and stem = 1; formic acid in leaves = 1; saponin in leaves = 1; amygdalin in stem = 1.

12

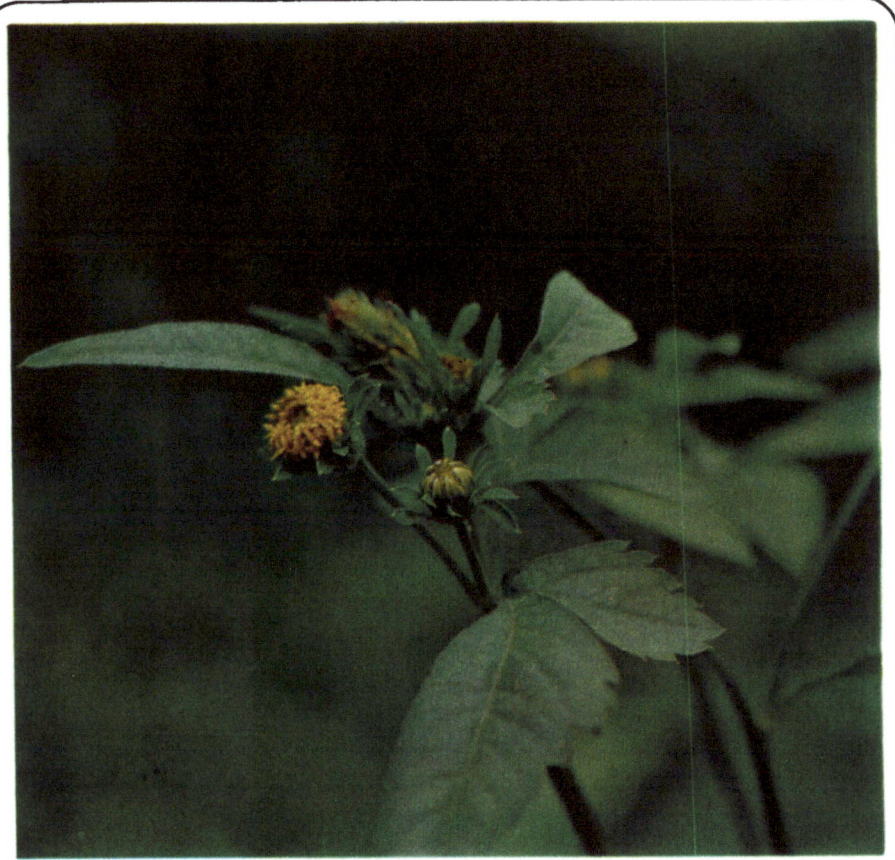

COMPOSITAE
Bidens pilosa L.
Burburtak, puriket (Ilk.); *dadayem* (Batanes Is.); *ang-nguad*
(Beng.); beggar-ticks, spanish needles, railway daisy, blackjack (Engl.).

An erect, branched, more or less hairy herb 0.2 to 1.5 m in height. The leaves are up to 15 cm in length, the upper ones usually much smaller. They are once or twice pinnately divided. The flowering heads are about 8 mm long, the disc flowers brown or yellowish, the ray ones yellow or nearly white. The seeds are black, 1 to 1.5 cm. long, with four projections at the apex.

Very common and widely distributed in the Philippines.

An infusion of the plant is used for the treatment of dysentery. Warmed juice of the fresh plant is used as drops for earache; for conjunctivitis; and as a styptic on wounds. Leaves are used as an enema for abdominal troubles. An infusion of the leaf and root is a colic remedy. This plant appears to have reduced the incidence of goiter in communities where it is eaten as vegetable.

Tannin in leaves = 1-2, stem = 1; saponin in leaves and stem = 1; sulfur in flowers = 1-2.

13

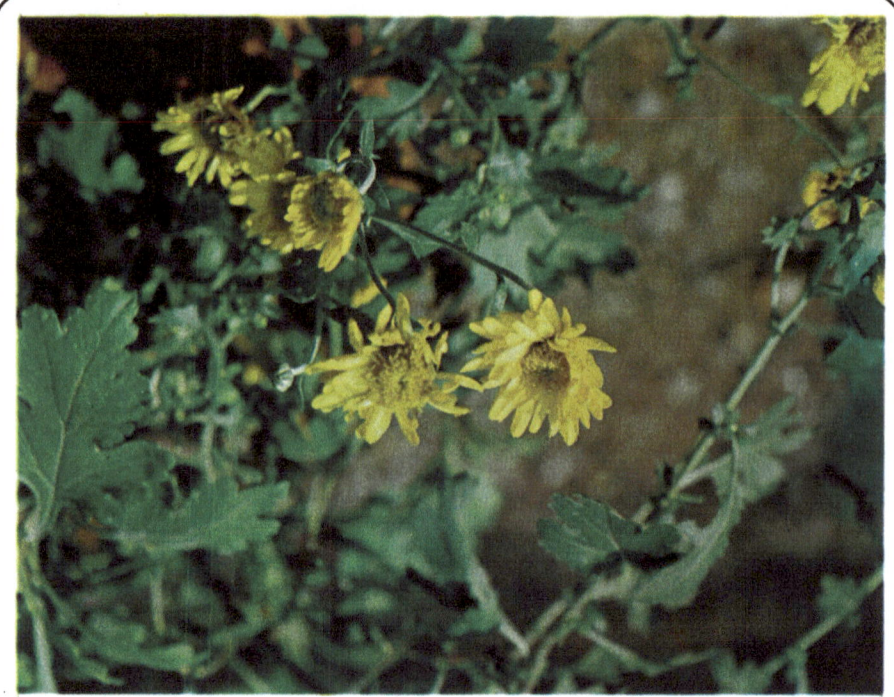

COMPOSITAE

Chrysanthemum indicum L.

Dolontas (Tag.); *manzanilla, rosas de japon* (Sp., Tag.); *mansanilya-a-babasit* (Ilk.); Indian chrysanthemum or false chamomile, winter aster (Engl.).

An erect or ascending, somewhat whitish, hairy herb, perennial, aromatic, 30-60 cm high. Leaves thin, pinnately lobed, the lobes 2 or 3 on each side, ovate or oblong-ovate, sharply toothed. Flowers in heads; heads yellow, peduncled, corymbosely panicled, and 1.5-2.5 cm in diameter. Involucre bracts oblong or elliptic, as large as the achenes. Receptacle smooth or pitted. Ray flowers uni-seriate, female, ligule spreading, disc flowers numerous. Fruit achenes, very small, cuneate-oblong, somewhat compressed and grooved.

Widely cultivated for ornamental and medicinal purposes.

Infusion of the flowers is used as a remedy for intermittent fever, hysteria and monthly irregularities; also used as a carminative, tonic, sedative, and for hypertension. Leaf decoction is a remedy for colds and headaches. Decoction or infusion of the whole plant or flowers is given in bronchitis, whooping cough, rheumatism, for swellings, boils and abscesses. Flower heads in oil applied on abdomen for gas pain, as poultice, can be employed in fungal infections.

Tannin in stem and root = 1; calcium oxalate in stem = 1-2, root = 1; glycosides in roots = 1; iron, stem and root = 1; saponin in root = 1; fats, leaves and stem = 1.

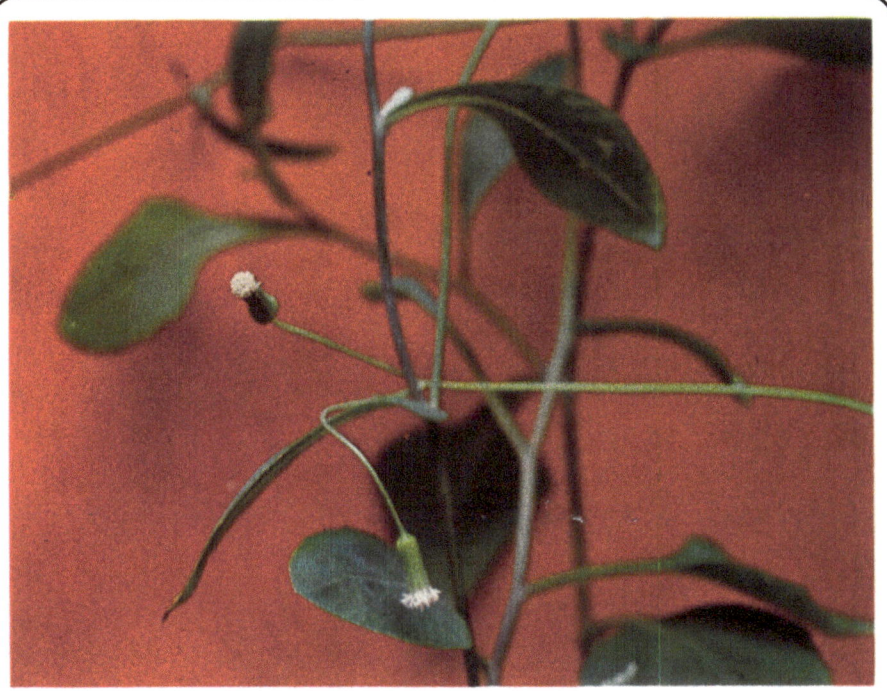

COMPOSITAE
Emilia sonchifolia (L.) DC. ex Wight
Tagulinaw, marsilanana, (Tag.); *lamlampaka* (Ilk.); *kipot-kipot, libua* (Bik.); *setim* (Bis.); *yayod-no-kangkong* (Batanes); red tasselflower, flores paint-brush, consumption weed, cupids paint, shaving brush (Engl.);

An erect or ascending, variable, glabrous or sparingly hairy, more or less branched plant, 10 to 40 cm high. Leaves somewhat fleshy, the lower ones lyrate-lobed or sinuate-toothed, 5 to 10 cm long, the upper ones much smaller and usually entire, all sessile and somewhat clasping the stems. Heads 12 to 14 mm long, long-peduncled, the flowering branches usually dichotomously branched. Involucre green, cylindric, somewhat inflated below, the bracts green, about as long as the purple flowers. Achenes about 2.4 mm long, narrowly oblong, ribbed, the pappus white, soft, copious.

Occasional in open grasslands, waste places; widely distributed in the Philippines.

Decoction or infusion of the plant is expectorant, and febrifuge. The plant is astringent, and is used as a vulnerary. The leaves and flowers are used as a styptic for cuts and wounds and for dressing ulcers. Root decoction for diarrhea.

Tannin in leaves and stem = 1; iron in leaves and stem = 1; pectic substances in leaves and stem = 1-2.

15

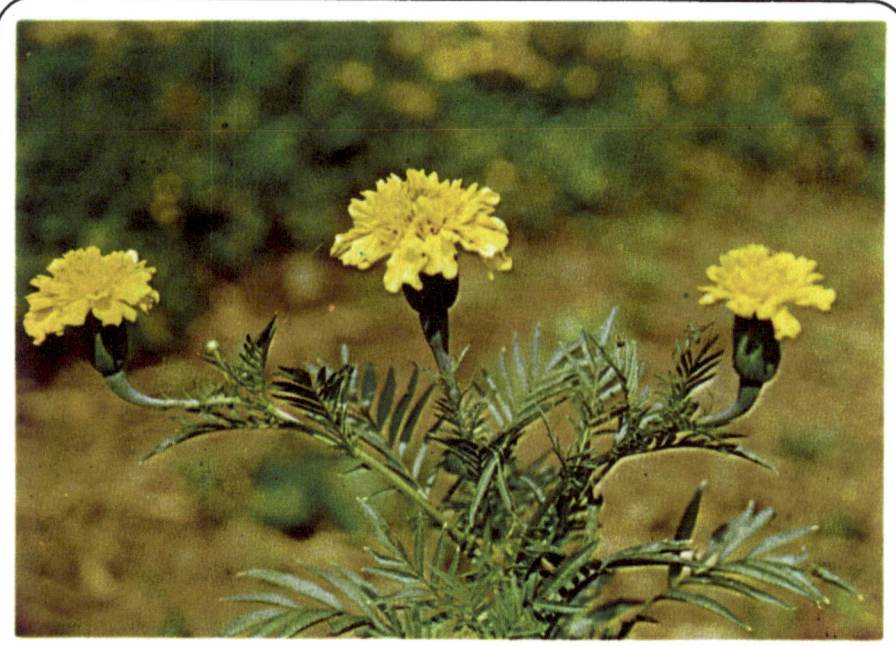

COMPOSITAE
Tagetes erecta L.
Amarillo (Sp., Tag.); *ahito* (Ilk., Tag.); marigold, African marigold,
French marigold (Engl.).

A rather coarse, erect, glabrous, branched, rank-smelling annual herb 0.4 to 1
m high. Leaves 4 to 11 cm long, very deeply pinnatifid, the lobes lanceolate,
coarsely and sharply toothed, 1 to 2.5 cm long. Heads solitary, long-peduncled, the peduncle thickened upward, 2.5 to 3.5 cm long, 2 to 4 cm in
diameter, the involucre green. Flowers pale to deep yellow. Achenes 6 to 7
mm long.

Commonly cultivated; in some localities spontaneous and naturalized.

Decoction or infusion of the plant is used in rheumatic pains, colds and
bronchitis. The leaves are used as an application to boils and carbuncles; their
juice for earache. Decoction or infusion of the leaves and flowers is carminative, diuretic and vermifuge. The flowers are employed externally in eye
diseases and in skin ulcers. The roots are laxative.

Sulfur in roots = 1-2; glycosides in stem = 1; fats in leaves, stem and
roots = 1.

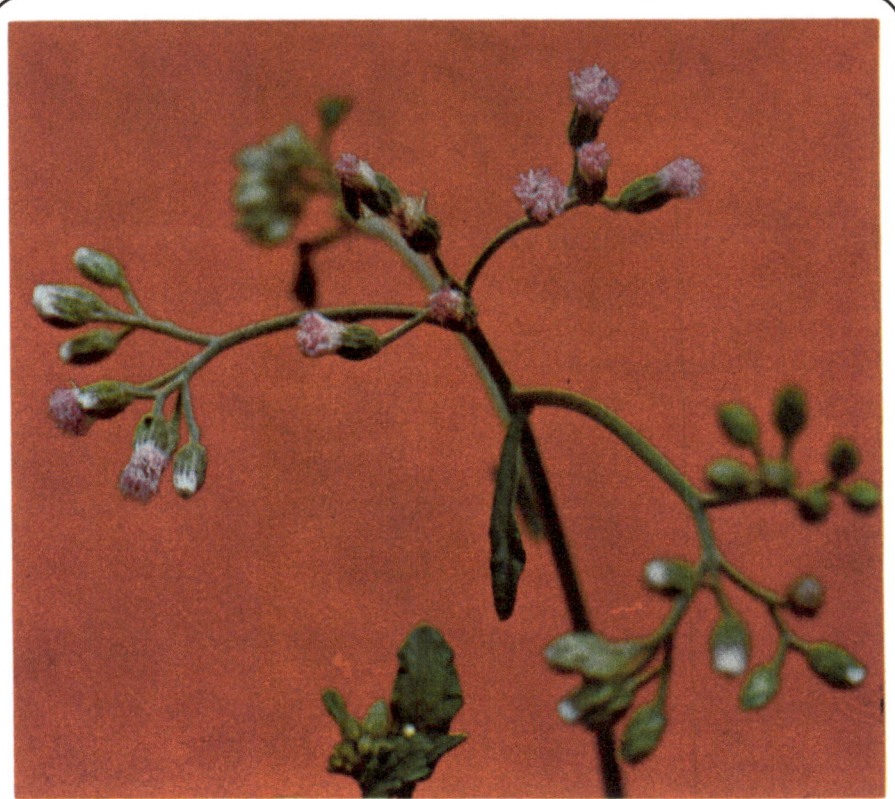

COMPOSITAE
Vernonia cinerea (L.) Less.
Tagulinaw, tagulinai, bulak-manok (Tag.); *agas-moro* (Ilk.); *magmansi* (Pang.);
sagit (Bon.); *kolong-kugon* (S.L. Bis.).

Erect, slender, perennial, branched, somewhat hairy, annual herb which reaches a height of 80 cm in the lowlands but maybe very small at high altitudes. Leaves are alternate, with short petioles, somewhat oval in outline, pointed at both ends, 2 to 6 cm long and with small teeth on the margins. Heads small, peduncled, in open lax corymbs, about 7 mm long, 2.5 mm in diameter, the flowers rather bright purple, about 20 in each head, twice as long as the involucral bracts.

Common in waste places throughout the Philippines.

Infusion of the plant is used in the treatment of cough, as a remedy for skin diseases and as a dressing on wounds. Leaves are made into poultice and used for headache. Decoction of roots is used for diarrhea and stomachache; vermifuge. The flowers are administered for conjunctivitis.

Tannin in leaves, stem and root = 1; calcium oxalate in leaves = 1, stem = 1-2; fats in leaves = 1-3, stem = 1-2.

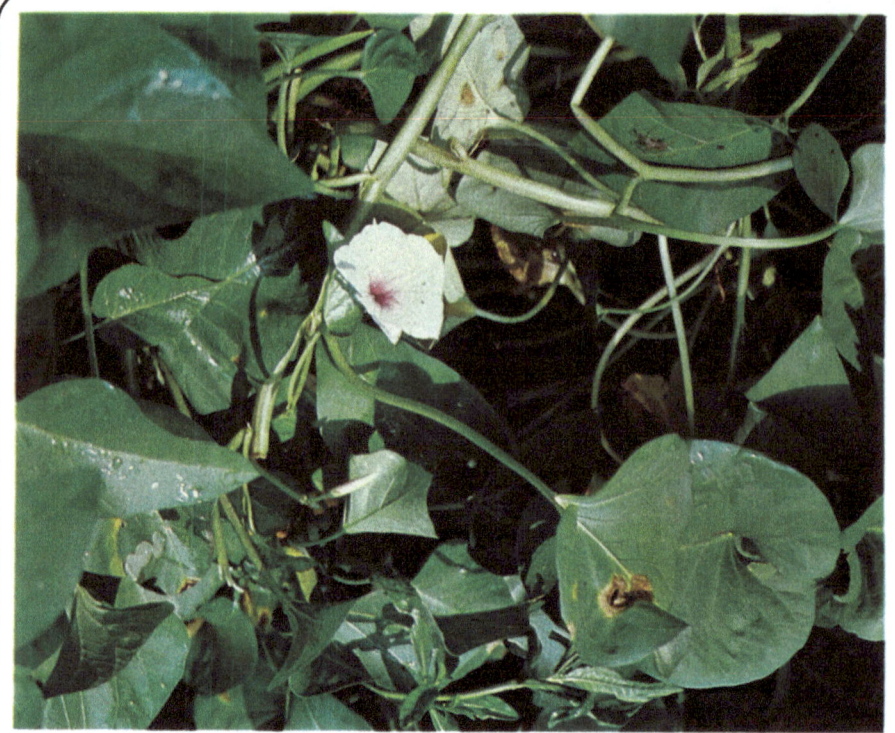

CONVOLVULACEAE
Ipomoea aquatica Forsk. (= *I. reptans* Poir.)
Kangkong (Bik., Tag., Pamp.); *galatgat, balangog, balangig* (Ilk.);
akangkong (Pamp., Bis.); *tangkung* (Zamboanga); potato vine, swamp cabbage
(Engl.).

An annual, glabrous, widely spreading vine, the stems trailing on mud or floating on stagnant pools, often thickened. Leaves oblong ovate, acute or obtuse, or slightly sinuate, angled or lobed, base cordate or hastate, 7 to 14 cm long, long-petioled. Pedicels axillary, erect, usually one or two flowered. Sepals green, 8 mm long, oblong, obtuse or acute. Corolla narrowly-campanulate, about 5 cm long, purplish; the limb nearly white or pink-purple, about 1 cm long.

Widely distributed in the Philippines in stagnant pools and open muddy places.

The tops are mildly laxative. The purplish kind contains an insulin-like principle and can be used as a cure for diabetes. The juice is employed as an emetic in cases of arsenic and opium poisoning. Buds are applied to ringworms.

Calcium oxalate in leaves = 1, stem = 1-2; tannin in leaves = 1, stem = 2; fatty substances in stem = 1.

18

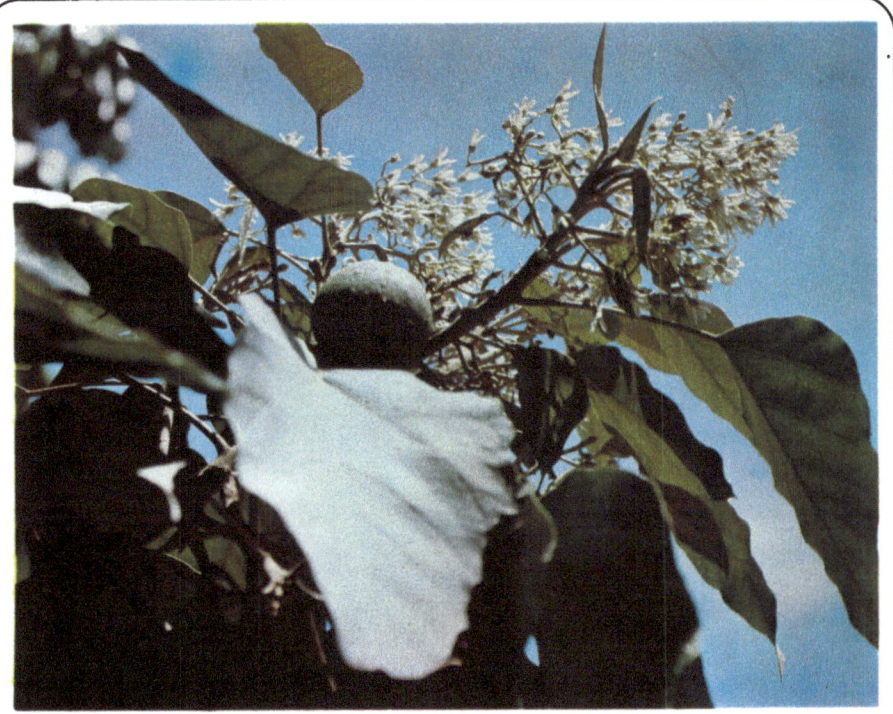

EUPHORBIACEAE
Aleurites moluccana (L.) Willd.
Lumbang-bato, lumbang, kalumban, kapili (**Tag.**); *rumbang, biao* (Bis.);
kami (Sul.); candle nut (Engl.).

A large tree, the younger parts and inflorescence pubescent. Leaves long-petioled, ovate to lanceolate, 10 to 20 cm long, acuminate, base acute, trun-cate or cordate, the margins entire or three to five lobed. Panicles 10-15 cm long, pubescent, many-flowered. Flowers 6-8 mm long, the petals obovate-lanceolate. Fruit fleshy, ovoid, 5 cm long, glabrous, containing one or two hard-shelled, oily seeds.

Common and widely distributed in the Philippines; a native of Malaya and Polynesia, now planted in most tropical countries.

The leaves, heated, are applied in cases of acute rheumatism. Kernels possess aphrodisiac properties. The juice of the nuts is anthelmintic. The nuts, soaked in oil and placed in the anus, relieves piles. The oil has a mild aperient action like castor oil; also used as a dressing for ulcers. The seeds are used as mild purgative.

Tannin in leaves = 1-2, stem = 2; saponin in leaves and stem = 1; calcium oxalate in leaves and stem = 2-3; sulfur, leaves and stem = 1-2.

19

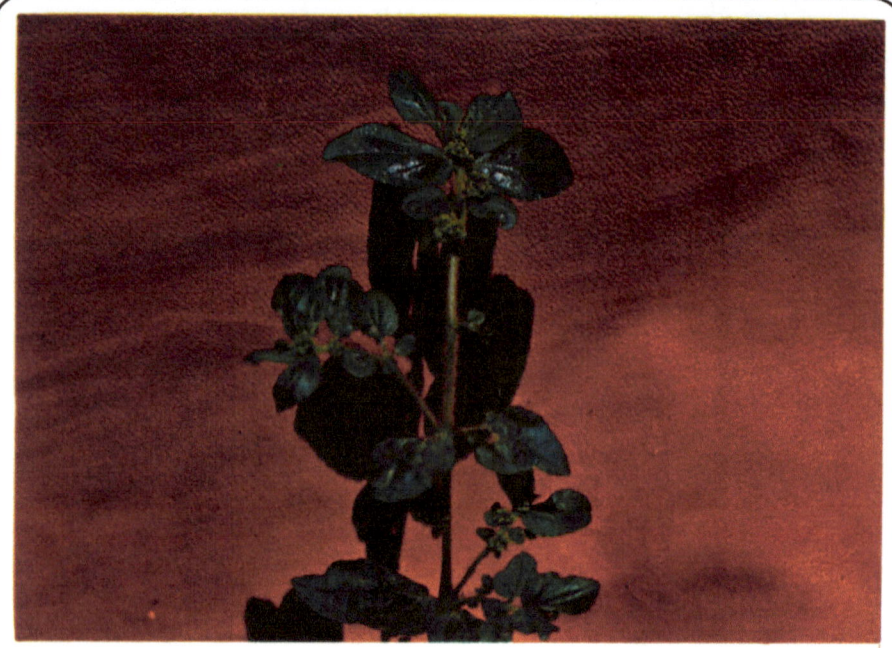

EUPHORBIACEAE
Euphorbia hirta **L.**
Golandrina, botobotones, botobutonisan, saikan (Tag.); *gatas-gatas* (Bis., Tag.);
malismalis, magatas, bolobotanis, sisiohan (Pamp.); *maragatas, botonis* (Ilk.);
pansi-pansi, soro-soro (Bik.); *tababa, bobi* (Bis.); *teta* (Bon.); *bambanilag* (If.);
asthma weed, snake weed, cat's hair, garden spurge (Engl.).

Annual, hairy herb, usually much-branched from the base, these branches
being simple or forked and ascending or spreading up to 40 cm long and often
reddish or purplish. Leaves opposite, distichous, elliptic oblong to oblong-
lançeolate, 1-2.5 cm long, toothed at the margin and usually blotched with
purple in the middle. Flowers are involucres, very numerous, greenish or
purplish, about 1 mm long and borne on dense, axillary, stalkless or short
stalked clusters or crowded cymes. Fruits are in capsules, broadly ovoid,
about 1.5 mm long or less, hairy and three angled.

Very abundant in the Philippines in waste places and open grasslands.

For asthma, burn and inhale smoke. Decoction of dried plant is applied
as wash for skin diseases. Infusion is used for stomachache and dysentery, as
bronchitis and asthma remedy; also used as cathartic, gargle and in the treatment of thrush. The root is a snake-bite remedy. The milky juice is dropped
into the eyes for conjunctivitis and ulcerated cornea. To stop local bleeding,
crush leaves, and apply on affected part.

Alkaloid in leaves = 1; tannin in leaves = 1-2, root = 1; calcium oxalate
in leaves, stem and root = 1; sulfur in leaves = 1, stem = 2; fats in leaves,
stem and root = 1; amygdalin in root = 1.

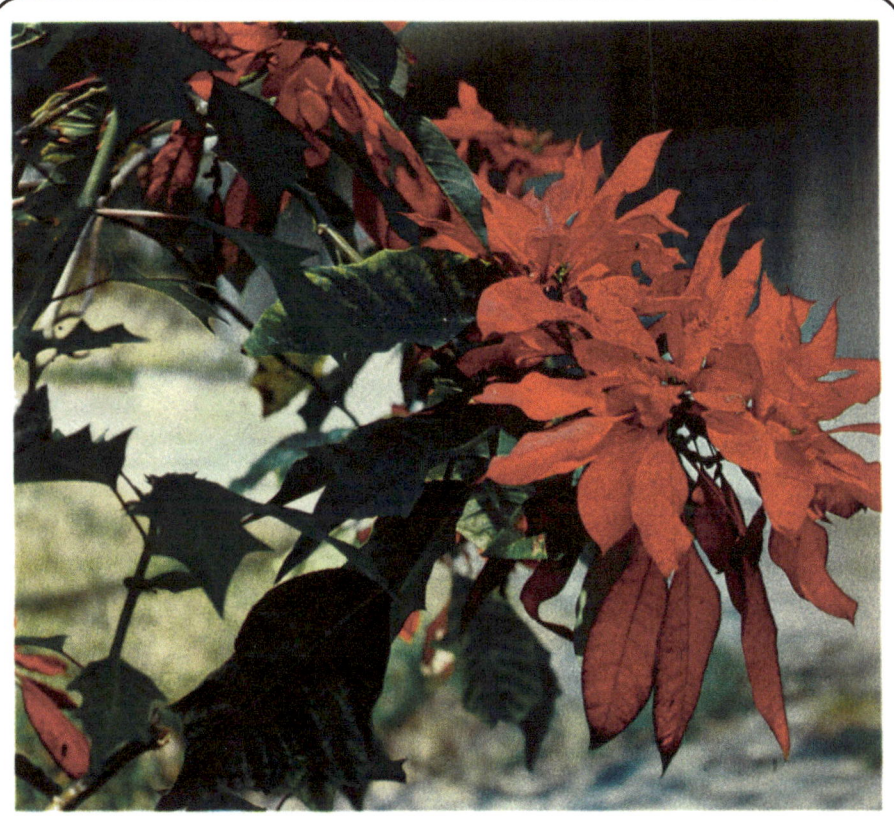

EUPHORBIACEAE
Euphorbia pulcherrima Willd. ex Klotzch
Pascuas (Sp., Tag.); eastern flower, christmas flower, poinsettia (Engl.).

Erect, sparingly and laxly branched shrub, 2 to 4 m high. Leaves are elliptic to oblong-elliptic or the upper ones lanceolate, 10 to 18 cm long, the lower ones entirely green, obscurely repand or slightly lobed, long-petioled, slightly hairy beneath; the upper ones, at time of flowering, uniformly bright-red. The inflorescence is terminal. The involucres are ovoid, about 1 cm long, the margins toothed, each with one or two large, yellow glands. The flowers are crowded, red.

Cultivated in the Philippines for ornamental purposes. It is a native of Mexico.

Leaves are applied as poultices for erysipelas and various cutaneous affections. Flowers in infusion are prescribed as a galactagogue. The plant is considered as an emeto-cathartic.

Alkaloid in leaves = 1; saponin in leaves and stem = 1. Sulfur in stem = 1; fats in leaves and stem = 1; amylodextrin in leaves = 1, stem = 1-2; formic acid in leaves and stem = 1; starch in stem = 2-3.

21

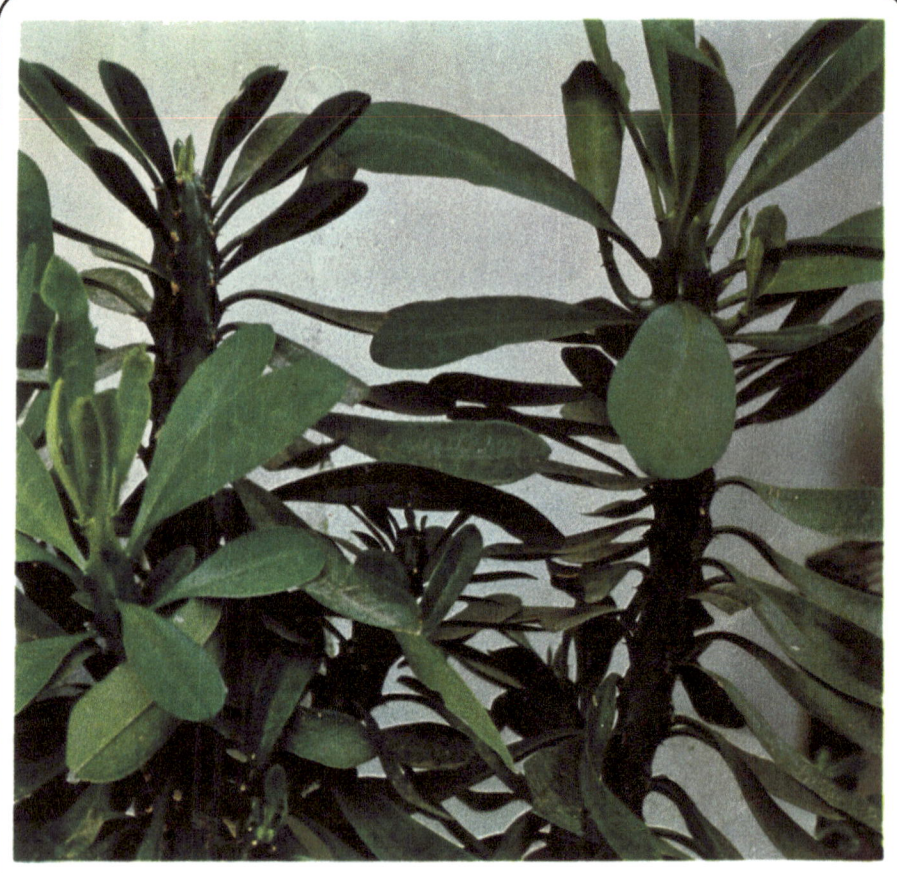

EUPHORBIACEAE
Euphorbia neriifolia L.
Soro-soro (Tag.); *lengua de perro* (Sp.); *bait, sorog-sorog* (Pamp., Tag.); *karimbuaya* (Ilk.); *sudusudu* (Bis.); common milk hedge (Engl.).

Erect, cactus-like plant. The fleshy oblong leaves are 5 to 15 cm long. The flowers (cymes) are short, solitary and green or pale yellow. It has spines and thickened stems.

Cultivated in rock gardens, probably introduced from Malaya.

The root is a snake-bite remedy. Latex is a remedy for earache, whooping coughs and asthma. It is also used as an insecticide, an antipyretic, drastic purgative and as an application to sores and cysts. Leaf has been used as diaphoretic.

Tannin in stem = 1; peroxidase in stem = 2, leaves = 1-2; calcium oxalate in leaves and stem = 1; fats, stem = 1; pectic substances in leaves and stem = 1; sulfur, stem = 1; starch in leaves and stem = 1.

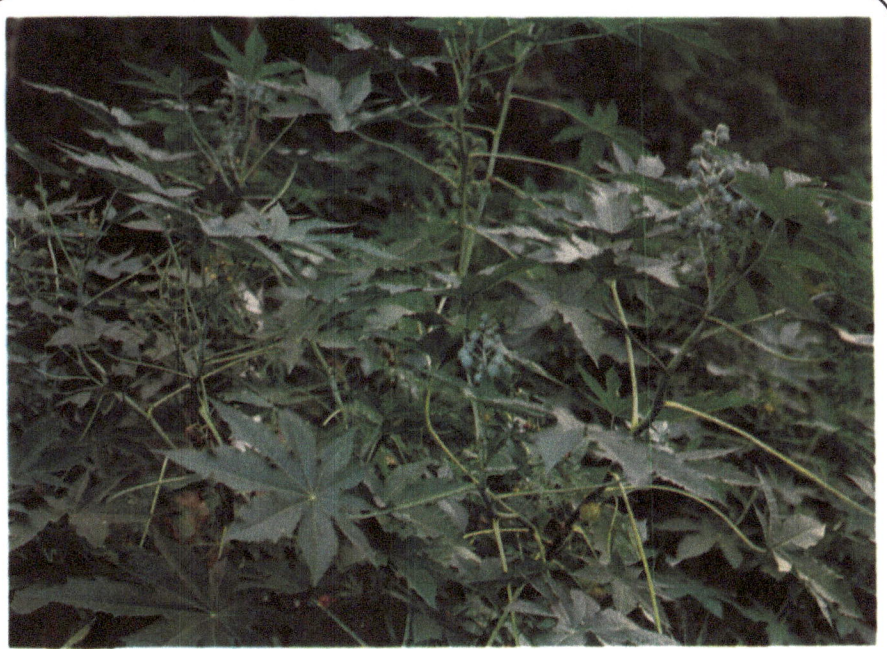

EUPHORBIACEAE
Ricinus communis L.
Tangan-tangan, lingang-sina, lansina (Tag.); *taca-taca, tawa-tawa, taua-taua sina* (Ilk.); *tangan-tangan, hawa* (Sul.); *casla* (Bis.); *tan-tangan* (Bik.); *katana* (Iv., Bon.); *gatlaoua* (If.); castor oil plant, castor bean (Engl.).

Shrub-like herb, stems 4-12 ft tall, branched, green to reddish or purple, leaves alternate, simple, long stalked, 20 to 60 cm wide and palmately lobed with 5-11 long lobes which are toothed on the margins, green, or reddish; fruits oval, green or red and covered with fleshy spines, seeds three per capsule, about $1/2 - 3/4$ in. across, elliptical, glossy, black or white or usually mottled with gray, black, brown or white.

Found in open waste places near settled areas throughout the Philippines.

Bark is used as dressing for wounds and sores. Leaf is applied to the head to relieve headache; pounded, it is commonly used as a poultice for skin ulcers, boils and over the breast for milk stimulation; is said to be an emmenagogue and also useful as a local application in rheumatism. Root is a remedy for abdominal pains and diarrhea; while the root-bark is said to be purgative. Dried root is used as a febrifuge and in the treatment of jaundice and nervous disorders. Oil obtained from pounded roasted seed is used for hemorrhoids and for various cutaneous complaints such as ringworm, etc.

Tannin in stem = 2-3, leaves = 2; calcium oxalate in stem = 2-3, leaves = 1-2; saponin, stem = 1; peroxidase, stem = 1-3; iron, stem = 1.

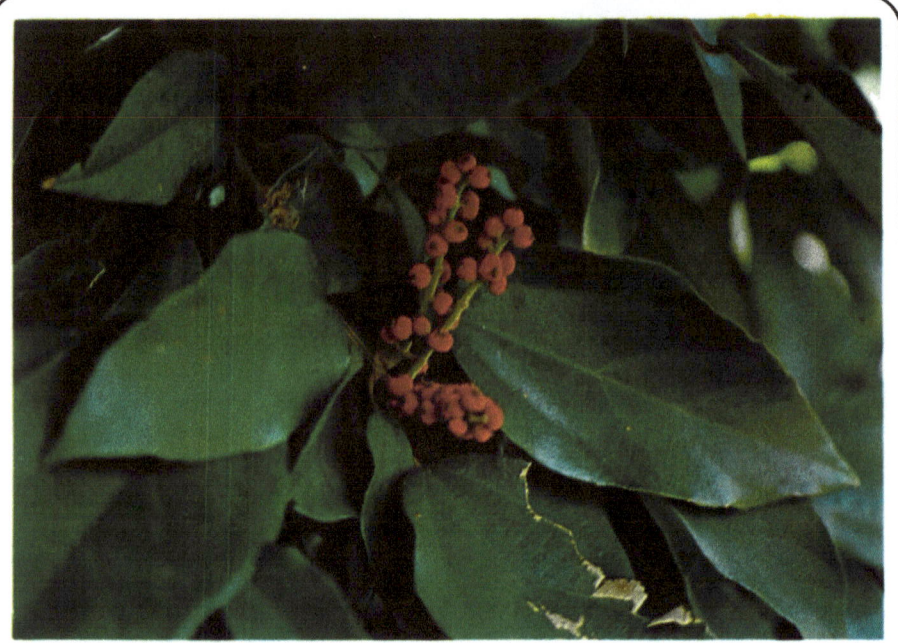

EUPHORBIACEAE

Mallotus philippinensis (Lam.) Muell.-Arg.
Banato (Ibn., Ig., Tag.); *apuyot* (Sul.); *buas. pangaplasin* (Ilk.);
darandang (Tag.); *panagisian* (Neg.); *panagisien* (Ibn., Klg.); *panagisen,*
tafu (Ibn.); *sala* (Tag., Bis.); *pikal* (Sbl.); *tagusala* (P. Bis.); *tulula*
(Tagn.); *tagusala* (P. Bis.); kamala, Rottlera (Engl.).

A tree 4 to 10 m high, the branchlets, young leaves and inflorescence brown-pubescent. Leaves alternate, oblong-ovate, entire or sinuate, toothed, acuminate, 7 to 16 cm long, rounded, three nerved, with two glands on the upper surface which is glabrous, the lower surface somewhat glaucous, puberulent, with numerous small, scattered, crimson glands. Inflorescence axillary. Male spikes solitary or fascicled, 5 to 8 cm long, densely many-flowered, the flowers about 3 mm in diameter, the anthers with crimson glands. Female raceme solitary, 3 to 7 cm long. Ovary and styles with crimson glands. Fruit subglobose, 6 to 8 mm in diameter, unarmed, densely covered with red or crimson powder.

Found in thickets. Widely distributed in the Philippines.

For fungal infection of the skin, pound leaves or seeds and apply on affected areas. Anthelmintic. Root infusion for leukemia and enema, and muscle pain due to fever. Plant infusion for bronchitis, meningitis, and typhoid fever.

Calcium oxalate in stem = 1-2, leaves = 2; peroxidase in leaves and stem = 1-2; fats, leaves = 1; tannin in leaves = 1; stem = 1-2; saponin in leaves = 1.

24

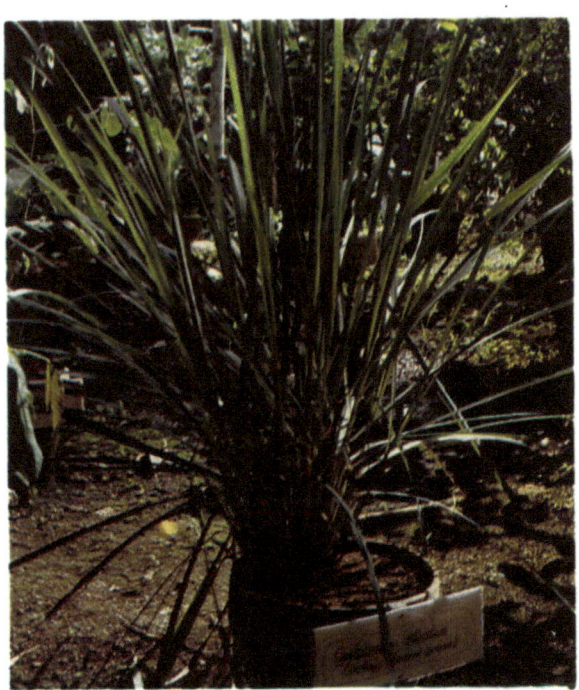

GRAMINAE
Cymbopogon citratus (DC.) Stapf (= *Andropogon citratus* DC.)
Tanglad, salay (Tag.); *baroni* (Ilk.); *belioko* (Bis.); *paja de meca* (Sp.);
lemon grass (Engl.).

A tufted perennial grass, the leaves up to 1 m in length, 1 to 1.4 cm wide, when crushed gives a strong lemon-like odor, scabrous, flat, long-acuminate, glabrous. Panicles 30 to 80 cm long, interrupted below, the branches and branchlets somewhat nodding. Perfect spikelets linear-lanceolate, pointed, not awned, about 6 mm long.

Frequently cultivated for its fragrant leaves which are used for flavoring food; widely but not extensively cultivated in the Philippines, not spontaneous, very rarely flowering.

Infusion of the plant is an excellent stomachic; with ginger and sugar, it is given as a diaphoretic in fever; also carminative and tonic, useful in cases of vomiting and diarrhea. Tea made from the leaves is diuretic and refrigerant. Leaves are employed for aromatic baths; applied to the forehead as a cure for headaches. The oil is antispasmodic and useful in flatulence; mixed with an equal amount of coconut oil, it makes a liniment for lumbago, chronic rheumatism, neuralgia, sprains and other painful affections. Root decoction with pepper is used for dysmenorrhea.

Tannin in root = 1; glycosides in root = 1; sulfur in root = 1; iron in leaves and roots = 1.

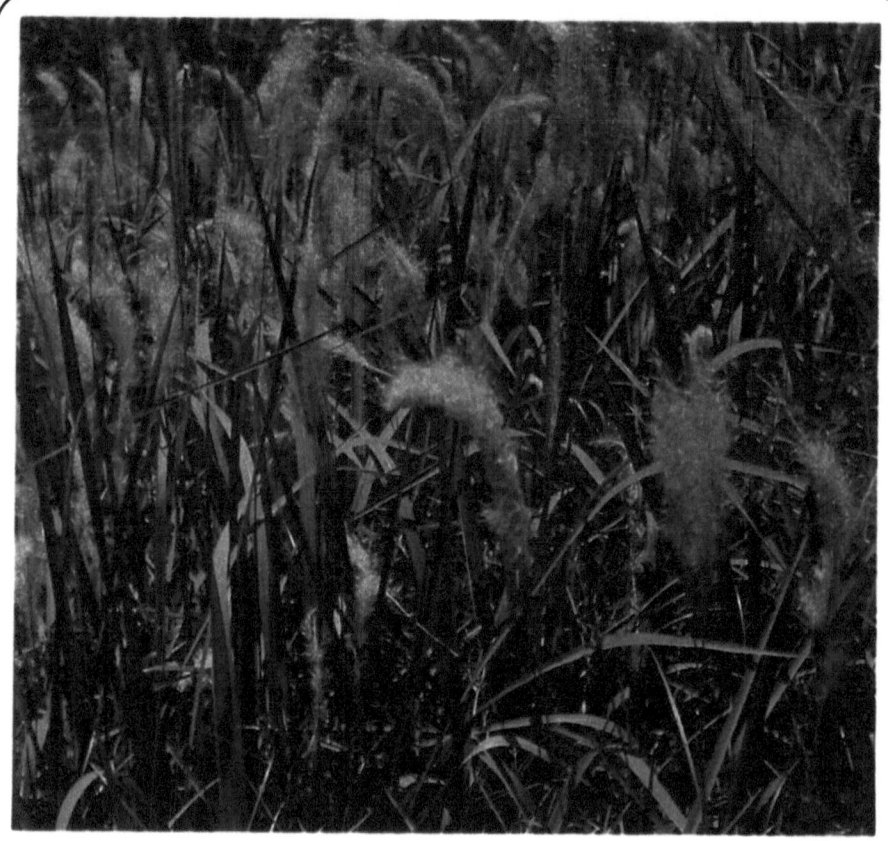

GRAMINAE

Imperata cylindrica (L.) Beauv. var. *koenigii* (Retz.) Dur. & Schinz.
Kogon (Ilk., Tag., Bik.); *ilib* (Pamp.); *gogon* (Bik.); *pan-au* (Ilk.);
parrang (Sul.); *gaon, bulum* (If.); *buchid* (Iv.); *gaon* (Ig.); *goon* (Bon.);
cogon grass (Engl.).

An erect grass, 30 to 80 cm high, the stems solid, rather slender, the nodes glabrous or bearded. Leaves flat linear-lanceolate, acuminate erect, 20 to 50 cm long, 5 to 9 mm wide. Panicles exerted, dense, subcylindric, spike-like, white, 10 to 20 cm long, 5 to 15 cm in diameter, silvery-silky. Callus hairs copious, about twice as long as the glumes. Spikelets 3 to 4 mm long.

It is found throughout the Philippines in open slopes.

Decoction of fruiting spikes is vulnerary; sedative when taken internally. Decoction of fresh roots is used in dysentery and indigestion. The roots and inflorescence are diuretic, restorative, tonic, astringent and antifebrile; also used for asthma, jaundice, nausea, dropsy due to weakness, and nosebleed.

Calcium oxalate in leaves = 2, stem = 1; tannin in leaves = 1, stem = 1-2; sulfur in stem = 1; fats in leaves = 1.

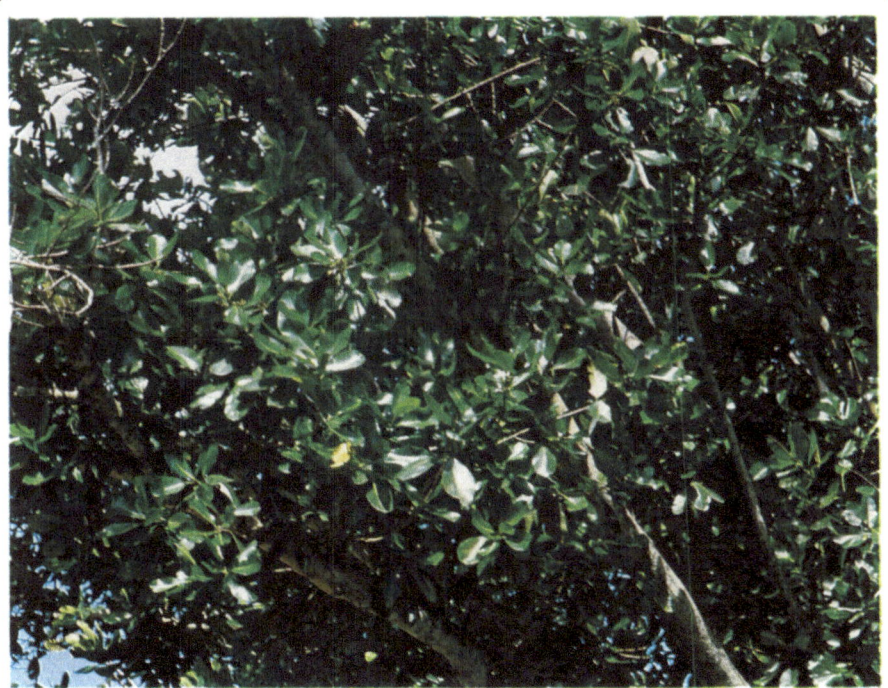

GUTTIFERAE

Calophyllum inophyllum L.

Bangkalan, bitok, bitong, dagkalan, butalaw (Tag.); *bataraw* (Neg.); *bitaog* (Ilk., Sbl., Pamp., Tag.); *bitaoi* (Pang.); *butalao* (Tag., S.L. Bis., C. Bis., Mbo.); *dagkaan* (Bag.); *dangkalan* (Tag., Bik., P. Bis., Mag.); *dingkalan* (Bik., Tag.); *langkagan* (Mag.); *palo maria de la playa* (Tag., Sul., Sp.); *pamitaogen* (Ilk.); *tambotambok* (Sul.); *vutalau* (Iv.); sweet-scented calophyllum, alexandrian laurel (Engl.).

A medium-sized or large tree, reaching a height of 20 m. Leaves coriaceous, shining, elliptic to obovate-elliptic, rounded, 9 to 18 cm long. Racemes axillary, 5 to 10 cm long, few-flowered. Flowers white, 2 to 2.5 cm in diameter, fragrant, the inner two sepals like the petals. Fruit globose, 3 to 4 cm in diameter.

Found along the seashore; throughout the Philippines.

Crushed kernels are applied on abdomen in gas pain, indigestion, colic, and on affected joints in rheumatism. Intramuscular injection of the refined oil have been used to reduce severe pain in leprosy. Infusion or decoction of the leaves is used as eye remedy. A gum resin from the bark is applied to wounds and old sores.

Saponin in leaves and stem = 1; tannin in leaves = 1, stem = 1-2; sulfur in leaves = 1, stem = 1-2; starch in leaves = 1, stem = 1-2; phytosterol in stem = 1.

27

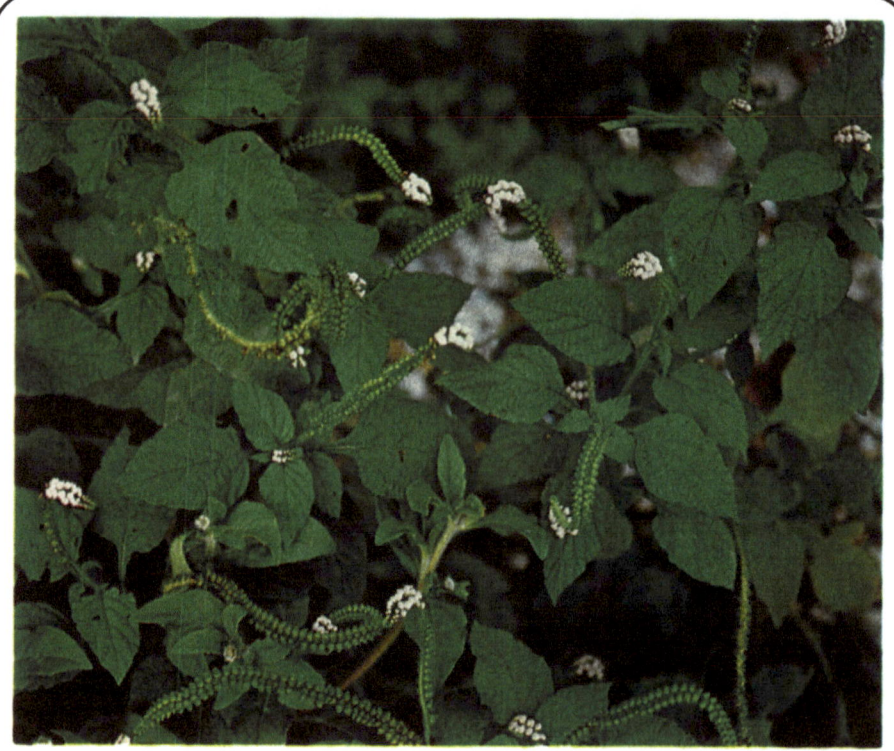

HELIOTROPIACEAE
Heliotropium indicum L.

Hikaw-hikawan, trompa elefante, hinlalayon, higad-higaran, kuting-kutingan, malakudkuran (Tag.); *buntot-leon* (Tag., Bik.); *kambra-kabra* (Bis.); pengga-penga (Ilk.); Indian heliotrope, erysipela plant, scorpion weed, wild clary (Engl.).

An annual, erect, branched, hirsute plant 15 to 50 cm high. Leaves opposite or alternate, ovate to ovate-oblong, somewhat hairy, acute or acuminate, base decurrent along the petiole, 3 to 8 cm long. Spikes terminal or, leaf-opposed, 3 to 10 cm long, curved; flowers all on one side, the lower ones opening first. Calyx green. Corolla pale-lavender to nearly white, about 5 mm long, the limb 3 to 3.5 mm in diameter. Fruit 4 to 5 mm long, composed of two ovoid, beaked cocci or nutlets.

A common weed in waste places; throughout the Philippines.

Decoction of leaves, antiscabious. Juice of the leaves is used as an application on wounds, sores, boils and on face pimples. Concentrated decoction may also be used as an external wash over affected area. Decoction of dried roots or flowers is emmenagogue. Decoction of the plants is used for cough and asthma. Juice of leaves is used as eye drops for conjunctivitis.

Alkaloid in leaves and stem = 1; calcium oxalate in stem = 1.

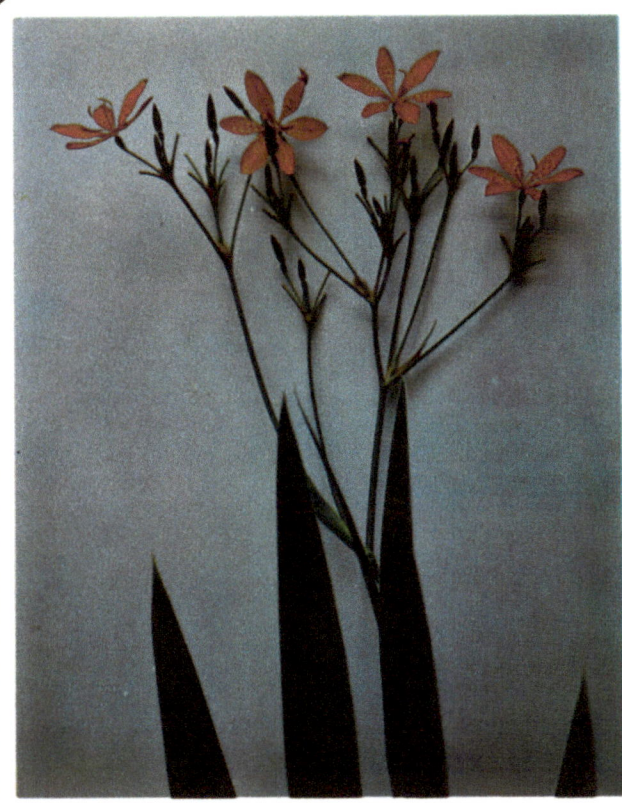

IRIDACEAE
Belamcanda chinensis (L.) DC.
Palma, abanico (Tag., Sp.); *abaniko* (Tag.); black berry-lily,
leopard lily (Engl.).

Erect, tufted, glabrous, 0.5 to 1.5 m high. Leaves two-ranked, strongly imbricated, crowded, narrowly lanceolate, acuminate, ascending, vertical, coriaceous, 40 to 60 cm. long, 2.5 to 4 cm wide, those of the stem equitant. Inflorescence terminal, erect, dichotomously branched, the spathes ovate-to-ovate-lanceolate, about 1 cm long, many-flowered, one or two opening at a time, 5 to 6 cm in diameter, the perianth-lobes spreading, narrowly-elliptic, tapered at both ends, yellowish outside, inside, reddish-yellow with darker spots.

Planted for ornamental purposes.

The rhizome is recommended as expectorant, deobstruant, and carminative; also added in tonics and purgative. It is given in pulmonary and liver complaints and for purifying the blood.

Calcium oxalate in leaves = 2; roots = 1-2, rhizome = 1; saponin in leaves = 1; tannin in roots and rhizome = 1; fats in leaves = 1, roots = 1-2, rhizome = 1.

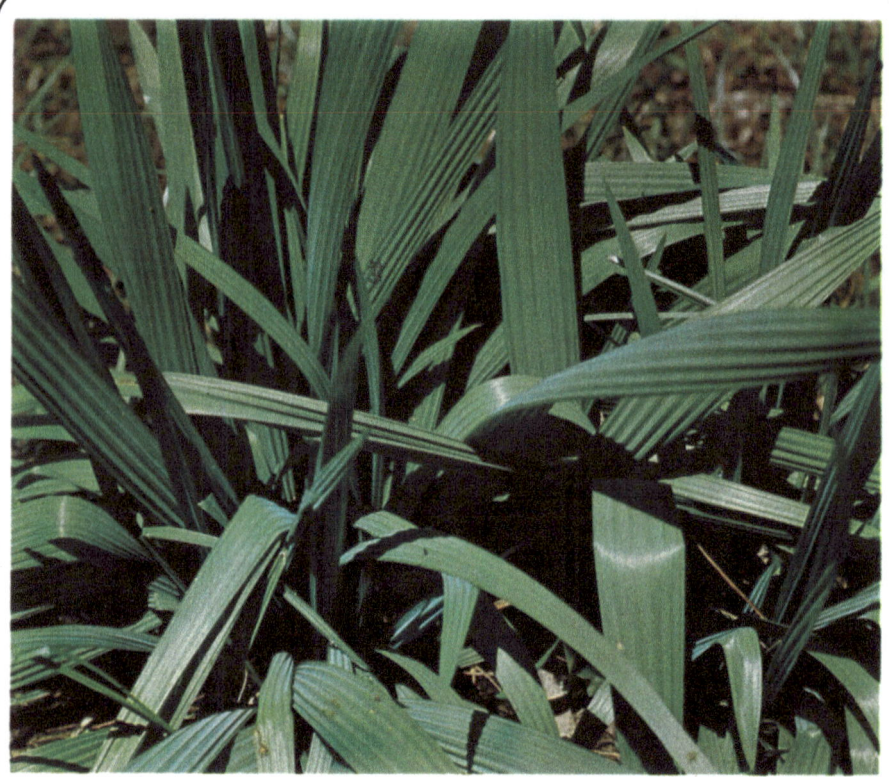

IRIDACEAE
Eleutherine palmifolia (L.) Merr.
Mala-sibuyas, rosas sa Siam, bakong-sa-Persia (Tag.); *hagusahis* (S.L. Bis.);
ahos-ahos (C. Bis.); *palmilla* (Sp.).

Bulbs about 4 cm long, ovoid-oblong narrowed at both ends, the outer layers thin, purple. Leaves lanceolate, narrowed at both ends, plicate, 2 or 4 from each bulb, 30 to 50 cm long, 1.5 to 3 cm wide. Scapes rather slender, as long as the leaves, green. Spathes 10 to 12 mm long, the outer two, green, the inner ones very much thinner, greenish-white. Flowers white, about 2 cm in diameter, the lobes obovate, spreading.

Occasionally cultivated, in and about some towns in the Philippines, sometimes spontaneous. Introduced from tropical America.

The bulb is pounded into pulpy mass and together with its juice applied to parts of the body of a person stung by venomous fishes such, as "sumbilang" to relieve the pains. Powdered roasted bulbs are rubbed against the belly to cure abdominal pains. Bulb decoction anthelmintic; macerated bulb topical for colic.

Tannin in bulb = 1. Starch in bulbs = 3, leaves = 1; calcium oxalate in leaves = 1; fatty substances in bulb = 1.

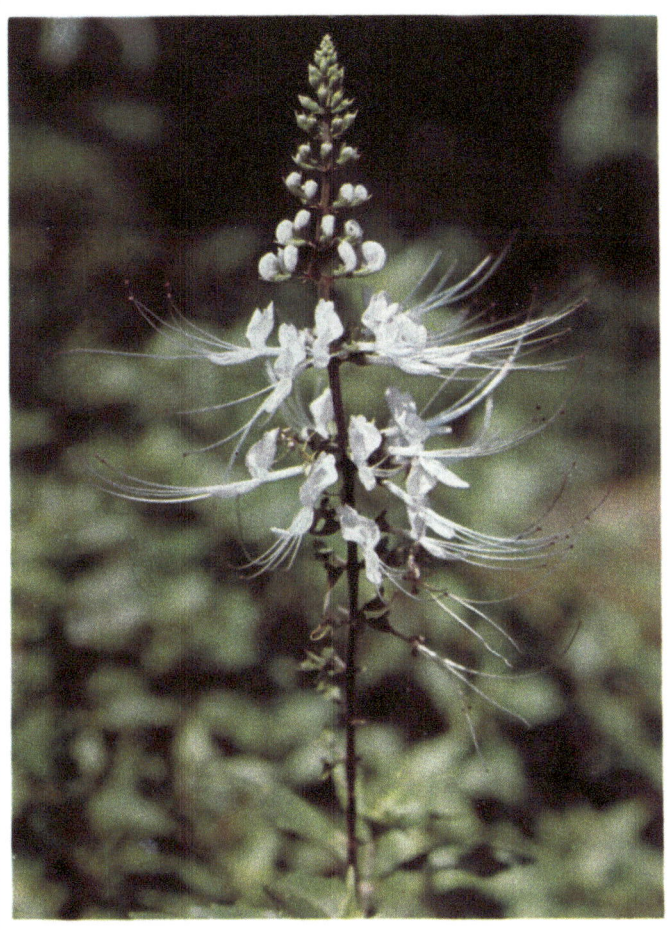

LABIATAE
Orthosiphon aristatus (Blume) Mig.
Balbas-pusa, kabling-gubat, kabling-parang (Tag.).

This is a slender, smooth or hairy undershrub 30 to 60 cm in height. The leaves are in distant pairs, narrowed into the stalk, ovate, 5 to 10 cm long, pointed at both ends, coarsely toothed at the margins. Flowers borne in very lax racemes. Calyx bell-shaped, with naked throat and two slender lower teeth. Corolla 2.5 cm long, smooth, white or purplish, very slender tube twice as long as the calyx. Nutlets oblong, compressed.

Found in thickets at low and medium altitudes.

Infusion of the leaves is used in the treatment of diseases of the kidneys, bladder and of the urinary organs. Leaves are also used for gout.

Tannin in stem = 1; calcium oxalate in stem = 1; sulfur in stem and root = 1; fatty substance in stem = 1-2.

31

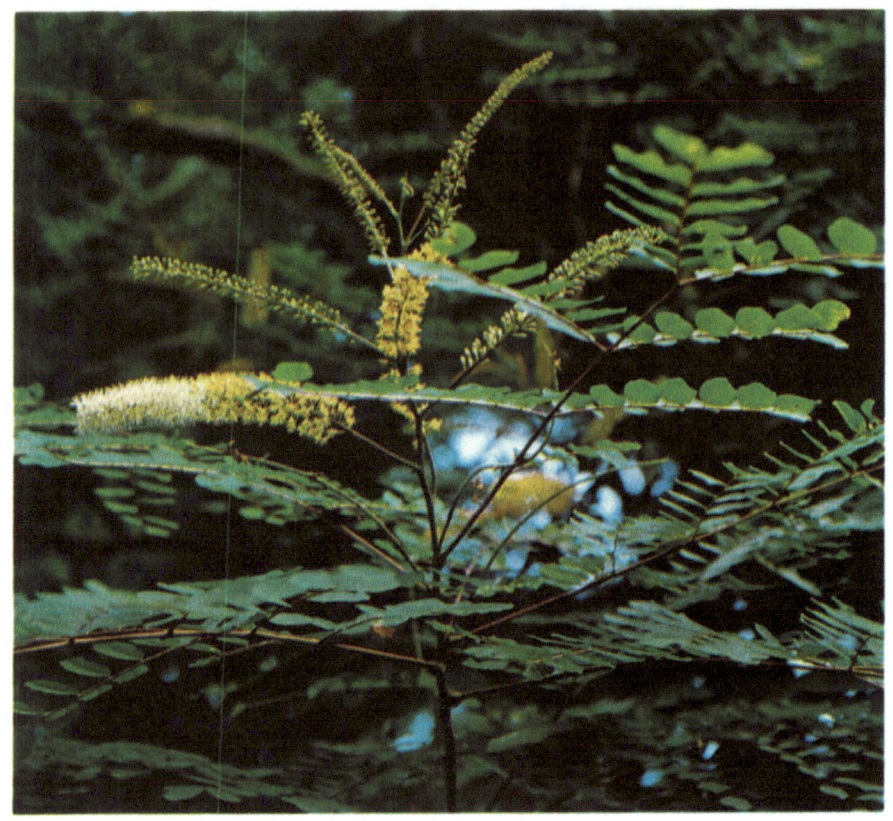

LEGUMINOSAE
Adenanthera pavonina L.
Saga, saga hutan (Malayan); circassian bean (Engl.).

A deciduous, erect, large tree. Leaves bipinnate, the pinnae are 8 to 12, opposite, short-stalked, and 10 to 20 cm in length. Leaflets are 12 to 18, oblong or elliptic oblong, evenly alternate, short-stalked, and 2 to 3.5 cm long. The racemes are 5 to 15 cm in length, simple from axils of the leaves, and panicled at the end of the branches. Flowers fragrant. The calyx small and bell-shaped with short teeth. The five petals are united at the base. The pods are linear, 15 to 21 cm long, and curved and twisted when opening. There are 10 to 12 seeds in pod, which are usually bright scarlet, shining lenticular, and compressed.

Cultivated in the Philippines as shade tree.

Decoction of the leaves is a remedy for chronic rheumatism and gout. Seeds are used for boils and inflammation. Leaves are also used as astringent and tonic for diarrhea and dysentery. The root is purgative and emetic. Bark is used for washing hair and clothes.

Tannin in leaves = 1, stem = 1-2; saponin in leaves = 1, stem = 2.

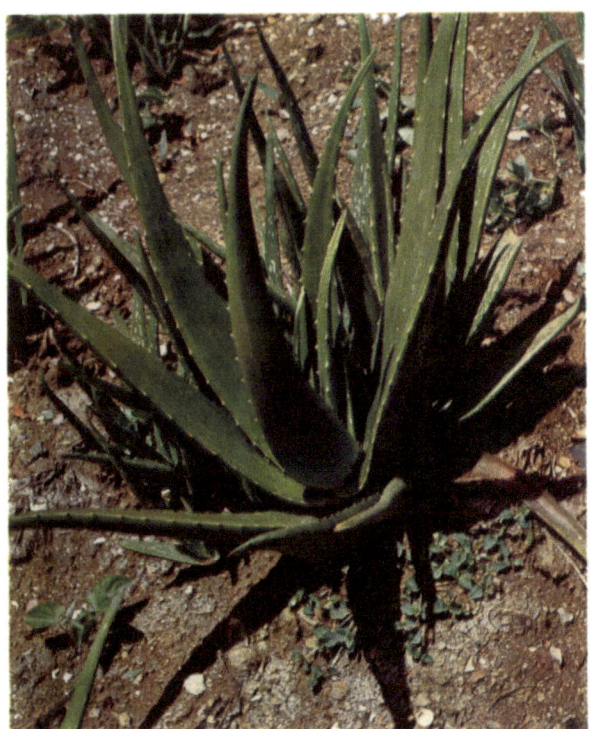

LILIACEAE
Aloe barbadensis Mill. ! [= *A. vera* (L.) Webb]
Sabila, sabila-pinya (Tag.); *dilang-halo* (Bis.); *dilang-boaia* (Bik.);
acibar (Sp.); aloe, curacao aloe (Engl.).

A short-stemmed herb cultivated both as ornamental and medicinal. The thick, sword-shaped leaves form a rosette immediately above the ground. They are 30 to 40 cm long, pale green with white spots and smooth except for weak marginal spines. The flower cluster (raceme), about 30 cm long, has a long stalk with distant acute scales. The yellow flowers without calyx are drooping, 2.5 cm long, tube shaped, tipped with short lobes which are curved outward. The capsule (fruit) bears angular seeds.

Commonly found in the Philippines as an ornamental.

Leaf juice is used for treating burns, abrasions and skin irritations; also purgative, vermifuge; tonic and remedy for kidney pains; cathartic; juice of leaves applied to the scalp prevents falling hair, and is said to be good for the complexion. Crushed leaves as poultice for contusions. Juice mixed with water is a remedy for indigestion and peptic ulcers. It is usually combined with other antispasmodic drugs; vermifuge; emmenagogue.

Tannin, leaves = 1; calcium oxalate, leaves = 2; sulfur, leaves = 1; fats, leaves = 1; iron in leaves = 1; formic acid in leaves = 1; glycoside in leaves = 1.

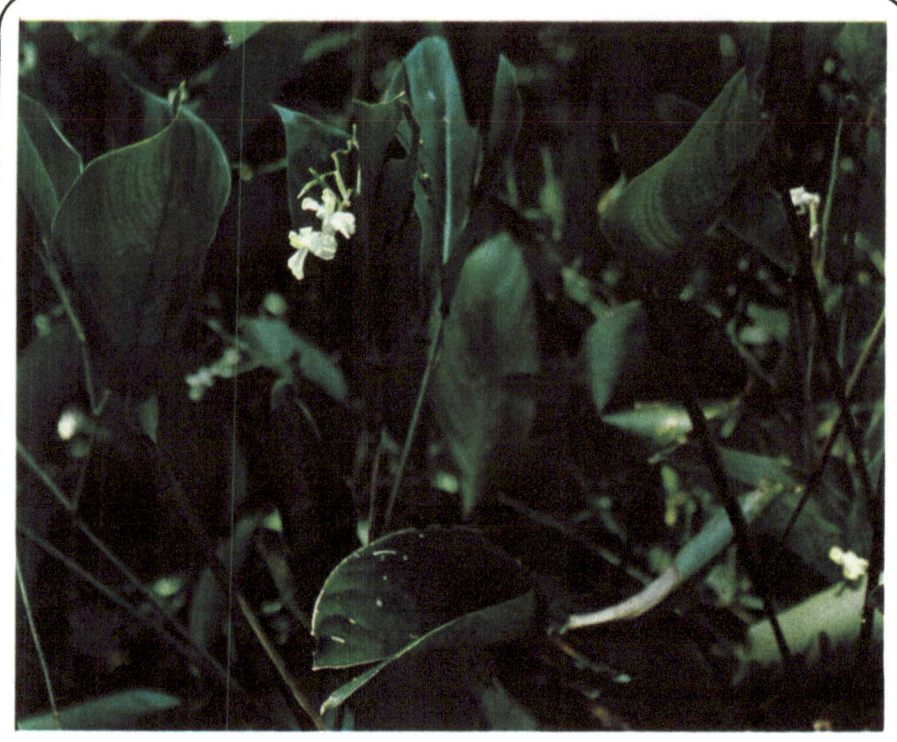

MARANTHACEAE

Donax cannaeformis (G. Forst)*K. Schum.*
Banban (Tag., Bik., Bis., Ibn.); *bamban* (Tag., Ilk., Bis., Sul., Mbo.);
alaro (Bis.); *baras-barasan, bonbon, manban, matalbak* (Tag.); *araton* (Gab.);
baban (Chab.); *bankolid* (Mbo.); *buaban* (Bag.); *daromaka* darumaka, garomaka,
lankuas (Ilk.); *matapat* (Ibn.); *mini* (Ig.); *ninik* (Iv.); *mamban* (Bik.,
S.L. Bis.).

A half-woody herb reaching a height of 1 to 3 meters. Bases of branches
somewhat swollen. Leaves usually rounded at the base and pointed at the tip.
Leaf bases very long and sheath the stem. Flowers white. Fruits rounded and
about 1 cm in diameter.

Common and widely distributed in the Philippines.

Decoction of the root is said to act as an antidote for snake-bite and in
blood poisoning. The young stems with ginger and cinnamon bark is swallowed for biliousness; juice from young leaves is given for sore eyes.

Calcium oxalate in stem = 1; sulfur in leaves and stem = 1; fats in
leaves = 1.

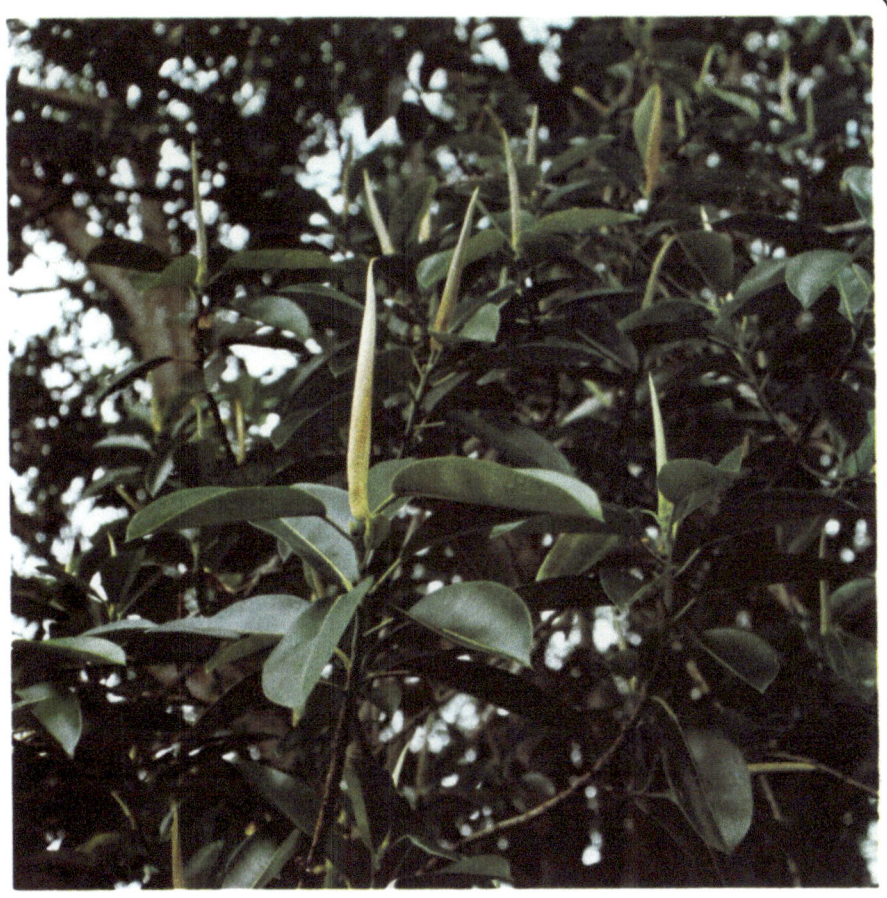

MORACEAE
Ficus elastica Nois. ex Blume
Balete (Tag.); Indian-rubber tree (Engl.).

A spreading, glabrous tree reaching a height of 10 m normally starting as an epiphyte, sending down numerous adventitious roots from the trunk and larger branches. Leaves very coriaceous, smooth and shining, elliptic-oblong, sharply and slenderly acuminate, 15 to 25 cm long, entire, the nerves very numerous, dense, parallel; stipulates deciduous, membranaceous, usually red, often as long as the leaves. Receptacles axillary, usually in pairs, sessile, smooth, greenish-yellow, about 1 cm long, oblong-ovoid.

Found in most large towns in the Philippines.

A decoction of the aerial rootlets is used as a vulnerary. The latex is administered to cases of trichuriasis. The bark is often used as astringent and styptics for wounds.

Calcium oxalate in leaves = 1, stem = 1-2; saponin in leaves and stem = 1; tannin in leaves = 1, stem = 1-2; fats in leaves = 1, stem = 1-3.

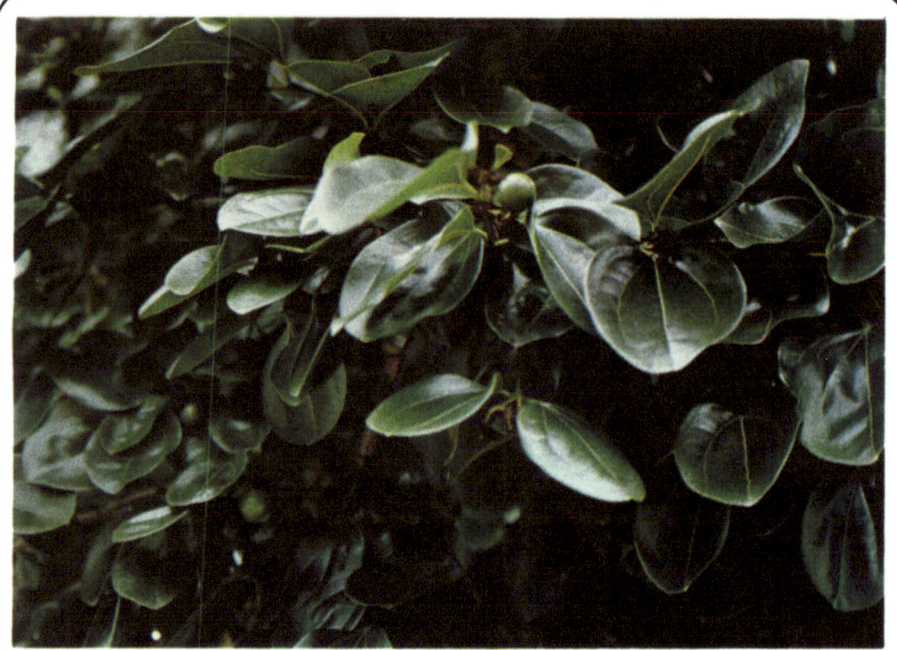

LONGANIACEAE
Strychnos nux-vomica L.
Nux-vomica tree, strychnine plant, poison nut, quaker buttons (Engl.).

A medium-sized, deciduous tree, 10 m high, with a straight, thick trunk. Leaves leathery, smooth, opposite, entire, shiny, broadly elliptic or ovate, 7.5 to 15 cm long and 6 to 8 cm wide, five-nerved, blunt or rounded at the base and pointed at the tip. Flowers greenish-white, numerous, small, and borne on small, terminal, hairy cymes 2.5 to 5 cm in diameter. Calyx small, with five teeth. Corolla tubular or funnel-shaped, with five reflexed, short limbs. Fruit smooth, indehiscent, orange-colored when mature, rounded, 3 to 5 cm in diameter. Rind is shell-like, pulp with two to five seeds embedded in it. Seeds are disc-shaped, nearly flat, 10 to 30 mm in diameter, 4 to 6 mm thick, shining, light silvery-grey and covered with closely appressed hairs. They are odorless but extremely bitter.

Introduced into the Philippines. It is a native of Sri Lanka, India and Burma.

The seed is nervine, stomachic, tonic and aphrodisiac; also a respiratory and cardiac stimulant. In excessive doses, it is a virulent poison producing tetanic convulsions. The powdered seeds are employed in a tonic for dyspepsia. The tincture of nux-vomica is often used in mixture for its stimulant action on the gastro-intestinal tract. It is used as a local anodyne in inflammation of the external ear.

Alkaloids in leaves and stem = 1-2, roots and seeds = 3; saponin in seed = 2; glycosides in seeds = 1; sulfur in seeds = 1.

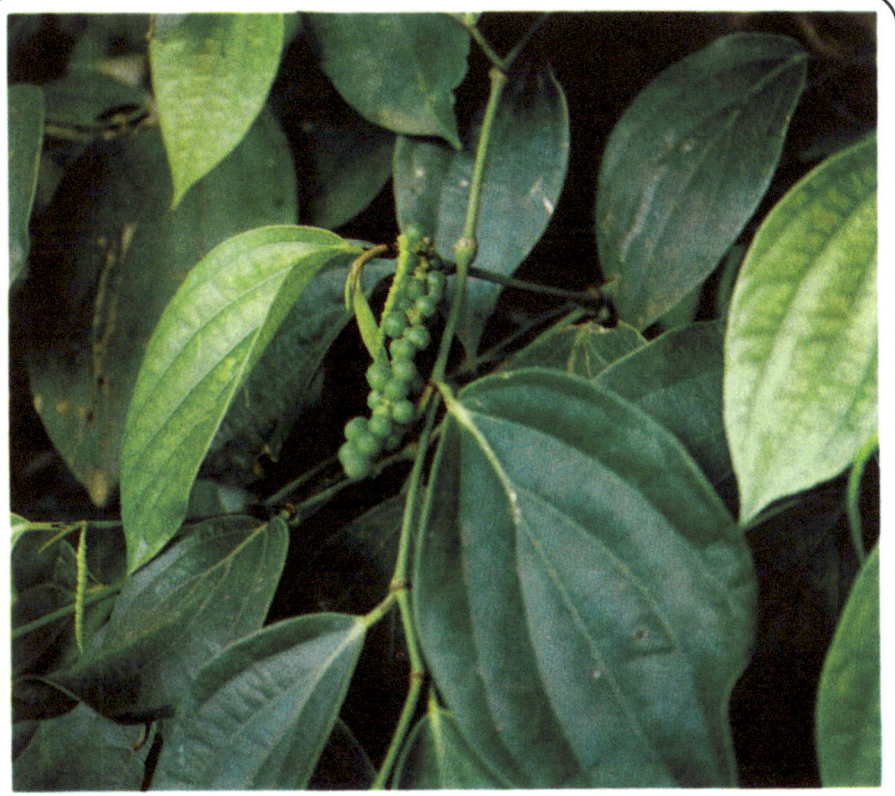

PIPERACEAE
Piper nigrum L.
Paminta, malisa (Tag.); *paminta* (Sp.); *pamienta* (Ilk.); black-pepper (Engl.).

A stout climber with smooth branches, 2 to 3.5 mm in diameter. Leaves somewhat leathery, broadly ovate to oblong-elliptic, 10 to 13.1 cm long, 3.5 to 8.1 cm wide with pointed, rounded or heart-shaped base, seven-plinerved, smooth on both surfaces. The rachis hairy. Bracts of the female cupular, receptacle short, whole, adnate without raised margins. The female spikes pendulous, 6.5 to 10.5 cm long. Fruits crowded, sessile, rounded, about 4 mm. long, 3 mm in diameter and with three or four stigmas.

Widely distributed in the Philippines.

Applied externally as a rubefacient and stimulant; used as a counter-irritant. Taken internally, it is carminative and stomachic; also used in cough, dyspepsia and flatulence. Decoction or infusion of pepper is used as a mouth-wash in toothache and as a gargle in various affections of the throat. Juice of the leaves is applied externally in scabies. Tonic, mild antipyretic; pepper mixed with oil has been said to be anti-fungal. It has also been used in vertigo, paralytic and arthritic disorders; in diarrhea and cholera.

Alkaloids in the fruit = 2; tannin in leaves = 1; stem = 1-2.

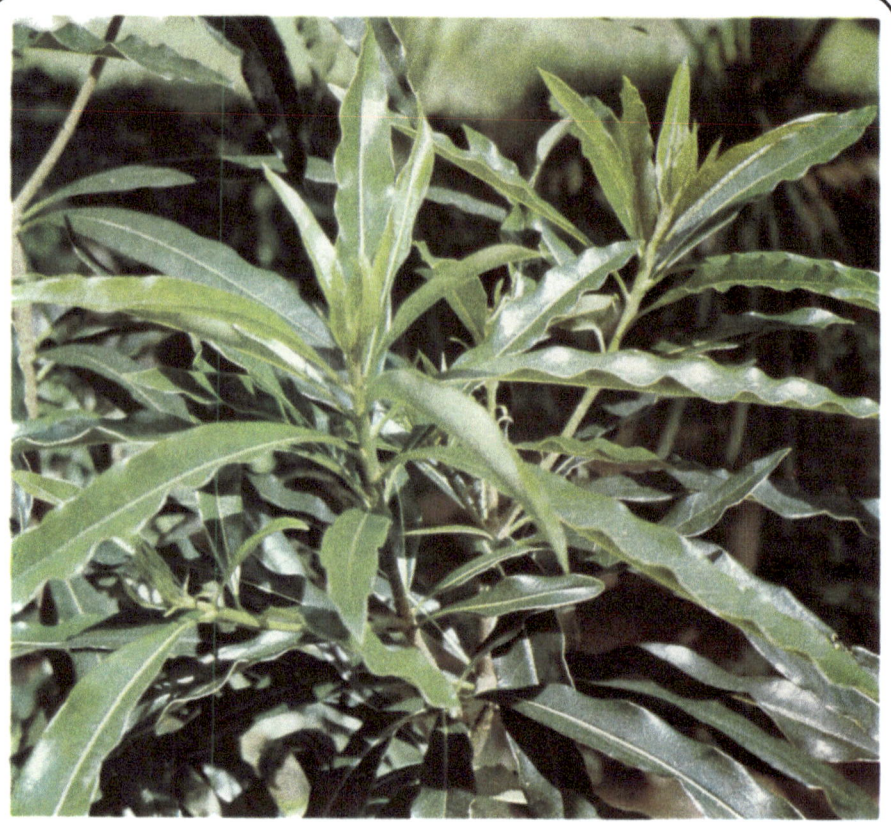

PITTOSPORACEAE
Pittosporum pentandrum (Blanco) Merr.
Mamalis (Tag.); *antoan, pangantoan, pangatoan* (C. Bis.); *basuit, oplat, uplai* (Ilk.); *darayan* (Tag.); *dili* (Gad.); *lasuit, pasgik* (Ig.); *mamali (Tag.); mamalis* (Pang., Tag.); *pasik* (Bon.); *taiu* (Sbl.); *balinkauayan, bolonkoyan, saboagon* (P. Bis.); *marabinga* (Tagb.).

A small tree 4 to 8 m high, glabrous except the inflorescence. Leaves lanceolate, gradually narrowed at both ends, rather slenderly acuminate, 6 to 15 cm long. Panicles 5 to 8 cm long, rusty-pubescent, rather dense, many-flowered. Flowers white, fragrant, about 6 mm long. Fruit subglobose when fresh, pale-yellow, 6 to 8 mm in diameter, resinous inside and with a strong, somewhat turpentine-like odor. Seeds brown, flattened, about 8 in each capsule.

Widely distributed in the Philippines.

Aromatic decoction brewed from the leaves is used by women in their baths following childbirth. Powdered bark in small doses is febrifuge, in large doses, a general antidote; also effective in bronchitis.

Calcium oxalate, leaves = 1, stem = 1-2; amygdalin in leaves and stem = 1; fats in stem = 1.

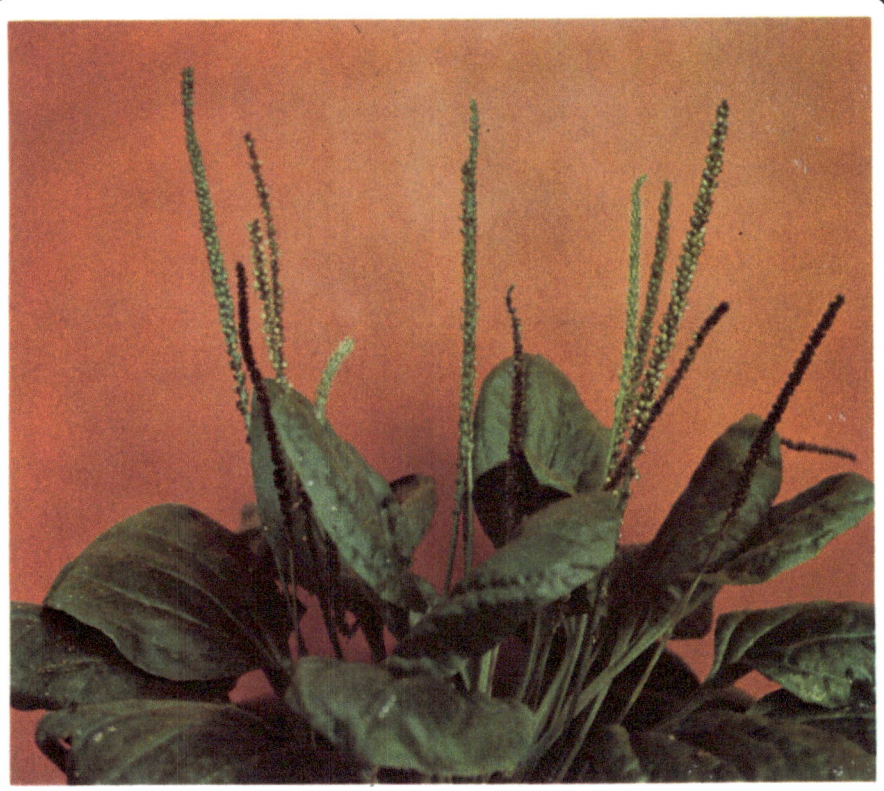

PLANTAGINACEAE
Plantago major L.
Lanting, lantin lanting haba (Tag.); *Ilantin*(Sp.); broad-leaved plantain, cart-tract plant, way bread, ribword, wild saso plantain (Engl.).

A perennial herb, stemless, with compact crown and fibrous roots. Leaves all radical (basal), in shape, long, ovate, entire, and when grown in rich damp soil they often become 6 to 8 inches in length. Blades are 5 to 9 ribbed and mounted on long-leaf-stalks. Flower stalks are usually longer than those of the leaf and bear a long, slender spike of many small, sessile, unattractive, green flowers, each flower is followed by a 2-celled capsule producing 4 to 8 small black seeds.

Found in cultivation and occasionally on waste lands at medium altitudes.

Used as poultice for boils, carbuncles and other skin irritation, as antidote for insect bites and diuretic. A watery extract of the seeds is given for whooping cough. For stomachache and malaria, the whole plant is boiled and the decoction is taken internally. Decoction of the leaves antidysenteric and vulnerary; also used as mouthwash for gum inflammation.

Saponin in leaves = 1; fats in leaves = 1; pectic substances in leaves = 1.

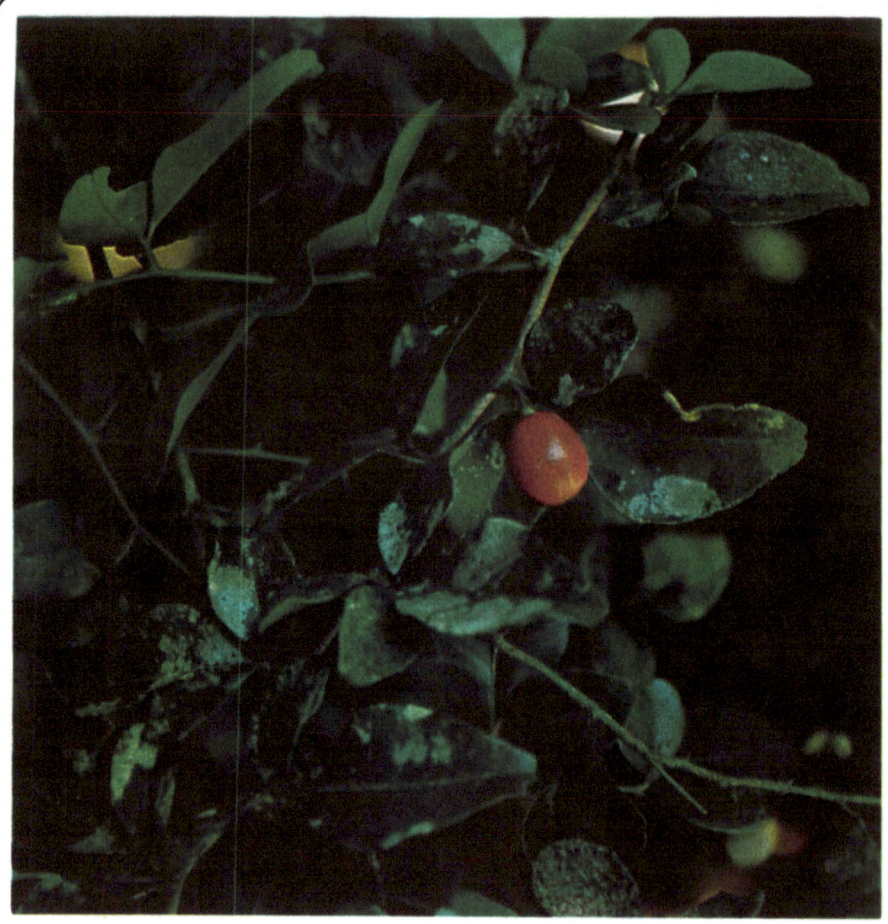

RUTACEAE

Triphasia trifolia (Burm. *f.*) P. Wills.

Limoncito (Sp., Tag.); *kalamansito* (Ilk.); *limonsitong-kastila, suang-kastila, sua-sua* (Bik.); *dayap, kamalitos* (Tag.); *tagimunao* (Neg.).

A glabrous shrub 1 to 3 m high, the spines in pairs, slender straight. Leaflets ovate to oblong-ovate, obtuse or retuse, crenate, the terminal one 2 to 4 cm long, the lateral ones smaller, the petioles very short. Flowers very shortly pedicelled, white, fragrant, about 1 cm long. Fruit ovoid, fleshy, red, edible, gland-dotted, about 12 mm long.

Widely distributed in thickets.

The leaves are applied to the body for various complaints such as diarrhea, colic and skin diseases; also used as aromatic bath. A medicine for diseases of the chest is made from the sweetened fruit.

Calcium oxalate in leaves = 1-2, stem = 2; fatty substances in leaves and stem = 2; formic acid in stem = 1; pectic substances in leaves = 1.

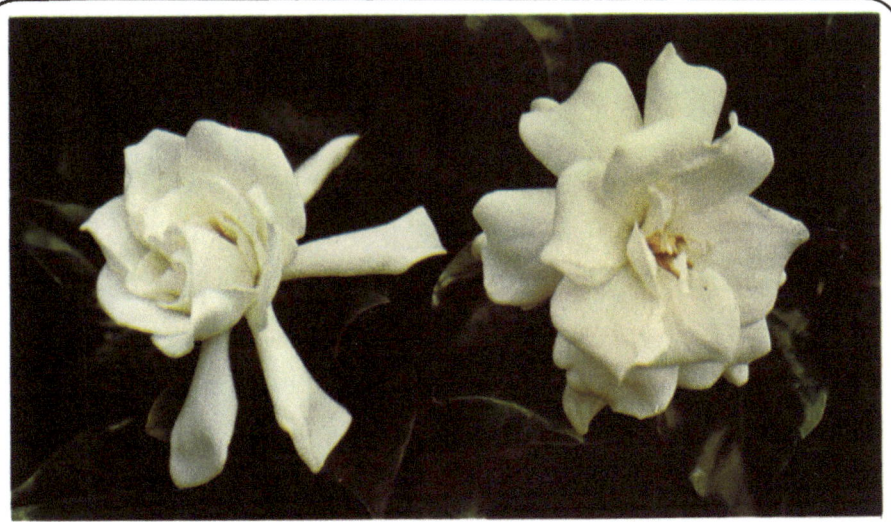

RUBIACEAE
Gardenia jasminoides Ellis
Rosal (Sp., Tag.); gardenia (Engl.).

Smooth, unarmed shrub 1-2 m high. Leaves elliptic-ovate, 2-6 cm long, narrowed and pointed at both ends, shining and short petioled. Stipulate. Flowers large and very fragrant, occurring singly in the upper axil of the leaves.
Calyx green with funnel-shaped tube and about 1.5 cm long, 5-angled, or
winged and divided into linear lobes about as long as the tube. Corolla usually
double, white but soon turning yellowish and 5-8 cm wide. Stamens as many
as the corolla lobes. Anthers linear, sessile. Ovary one-celled, style stout,
clavate, fusiform, or 2-cleft ovules numerous on parietal placentae. Fruits
ovoid or ellipsoid, 2.5-4.5 cm long, 1.5-2 cm in diameter, yellow, with 5-9
longitudinal ridges.

A common garden plant. Only the double-flowered form occurs in the
Philippines.

Leaves are applied as poultice to swollen breast, and for headache.
Decoction of bark is used in uterine troubles, intermittent fever, dysentery, as a
tonic and for abdominal pains. Decoction of roots remedy for flatulence
and dyspepsia. Flower infusion is emollient. The fruit has emetic, stimulant
and diuretic properties; externally the pulp is applied to swelling, burns and
scalds. Resinous exudation from the fruit acts as an antiperiodic, a cathartic,
an anthelmintic, alternative and as antispasmodic; externally, it acts as an
antiseptic and a stimulant; applied also to ulcers. The fruit is used in jaundice;
also antipyretic. It has been reported to have antifungal and anti-bacterial
action.

Tannin in leaves and stem = 1; saponin, leaves, stem = 1-2; calcium
oxalate in leaves = 2, stem = 3; sulfur, leaves = 1; nitrates, leaves and stem =
1.

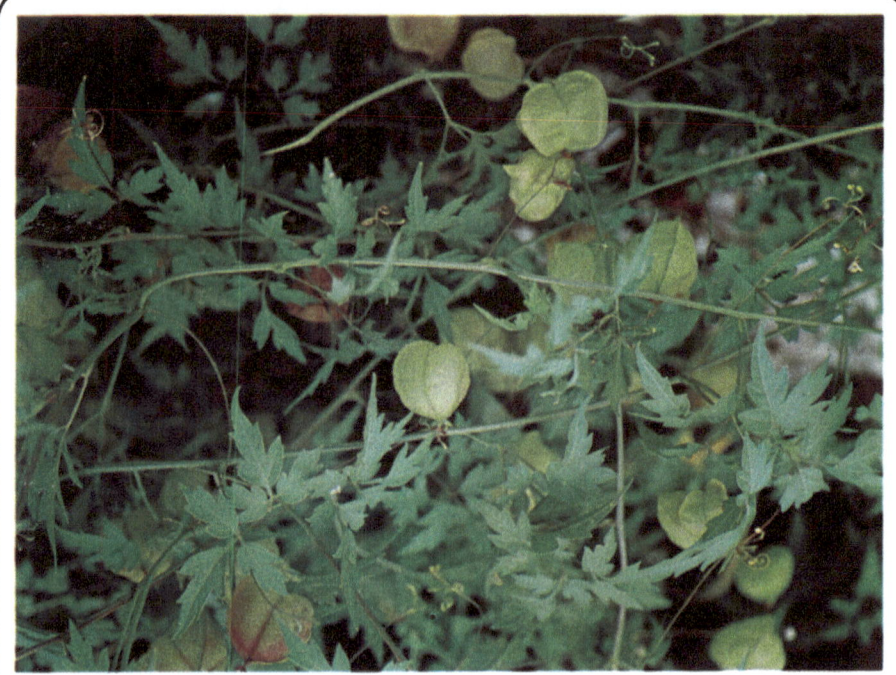

SAPINDACEAE
Cardiospermum halicacabum L.
Parol-parolan, bangkolon, lobo-lobohan, layaw (Tag.); *paria-aso,
paspalya* (Ilk.); *kana, ablayon, alalayou* (Bis.); *paltu-paltukan*
(Pamp.); balloon vine, leaved-heart pea (Engl.).

Slender, herbaceous vine about 3 m long. Its alternate, long-stalked compound leaves are divided into three branches, each branch has three leaflets.
Leaflets elongated, deeply-lobed with indented margins, the center lobe
sticking out farthest. The small white flowers are provided with a pair of
tendrils at the base of the clusters which function as support for climbing.
The bladder-like fruits filled with air are more or less triangular and ribbed.
They contain three round black seeds, each with a white heart-shaped spot at
the base, hence the name *cardiospermum, cardio* for the heart and *spermum*
for seed.

Found throughout the Philippines in thickets, waste places, etc., in
settled areas.

Infusion of the leaf and stalk is given in diarrhea and dysentery. The
leaf is irritant, rubefacient and emetic and is used in amenorrhea. The leaf and
root are used as a diaphoretic, as a diuretic in bladder disease and a remedy
for dropsy, rheumatism, nervous complaints and lung diseases. The root is
said to be laxative, and demulcent.

Saponin in leaves = 1-2; tannin in leaves and stem = 1; calcium oxalate
in leaves = 1-2, stem = 1; sulfur in stem = 1-2.

42

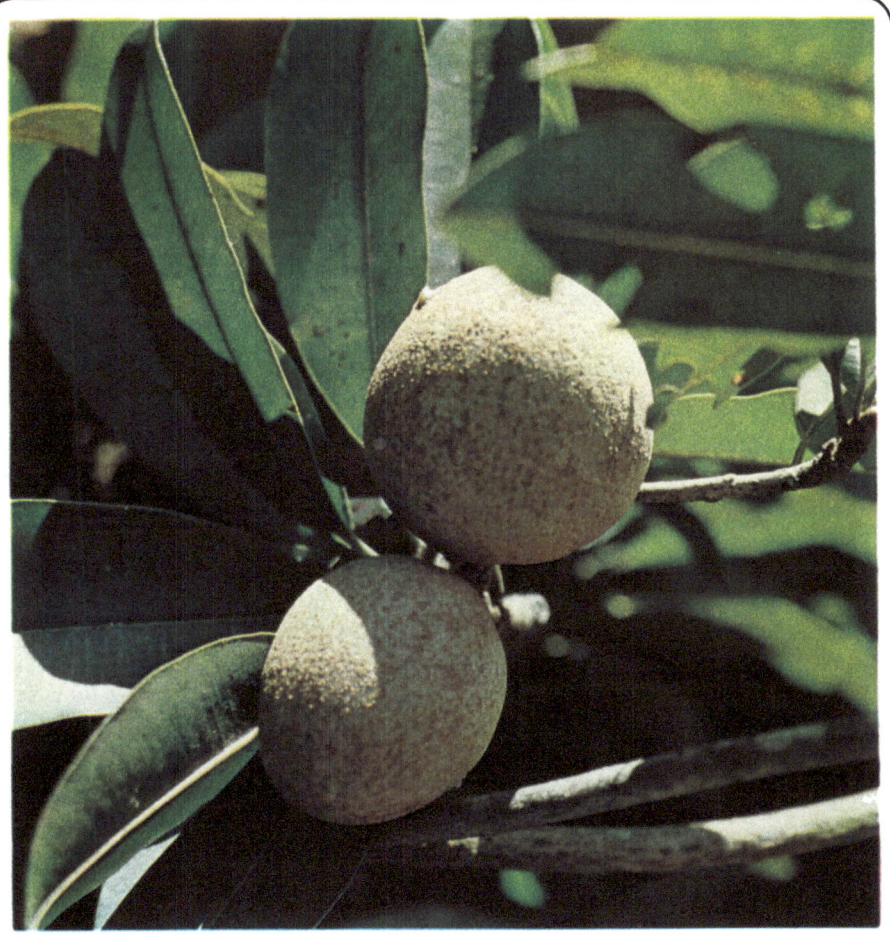

SAPOTACEAE
Manilkara zapota (L.) van Royen (= *Achras zapota* L.)
Chico (Sp., Tag.); *chiku tree, sapodilla* (Engl.).

A much-branched tree reaching a height of 8 meters. Leaves oblong to narrowly oblong-ovate, acute or shortly acuminate, base acute, 8 to 13 cm long. Flowers rusty-pubescent outside, 6 to 8 mm long. Fruit ovoid or sub-globose, brown, fleshy, 3 to 5 cm long, the soft rather sweet pulp edible.

Commonly cultivated for its edible fruit.

Decoction of bark is given for diarrhea and fever; also tonic. The astringent fruit is antidysenteric; prevents biliousness and febrile attacks. The seeds are known to be aperient and diuretic.

Saponin in leaves and stem = 1-2; tannin in leaves = 1, stem = 2; glycosides in leaves and stem = 1; sulfur in leaves = 1, stem = 1-2; iron in leaves and stem = 1; fats leaves and stem = 1-2.

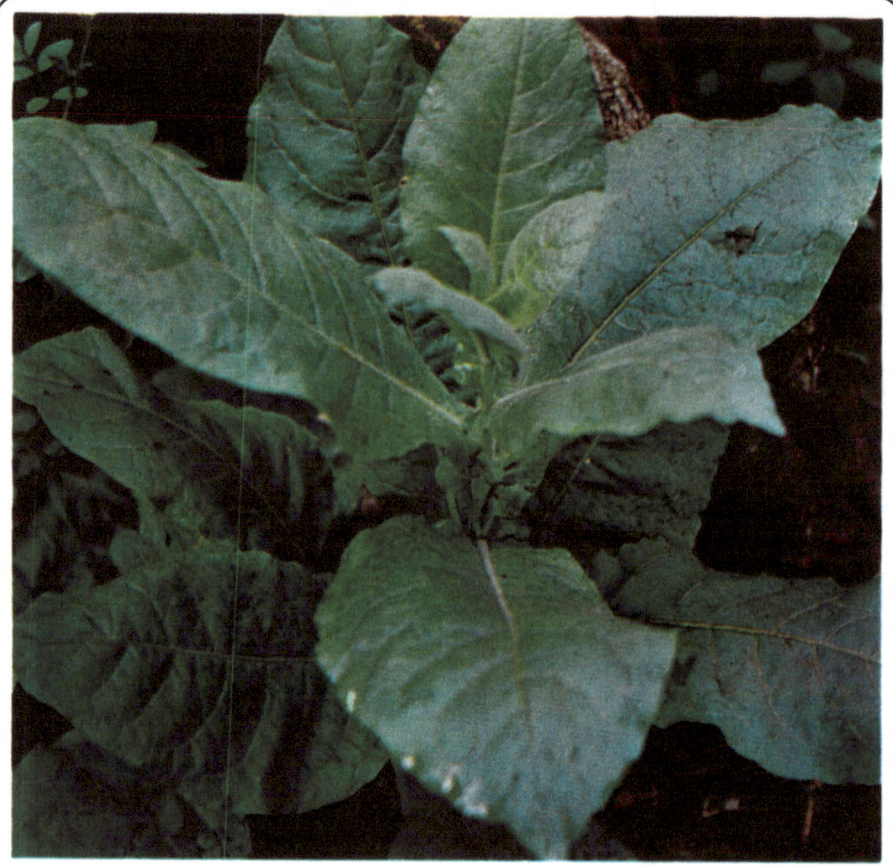

SOLANACEAE
Nicotiana tabacum L.
Tabaco (Sp., Tag.); tobacco (Engl.).

A coarse, erect, annual herb 0.7 to 1.5 m high. Leaves elliptic-ovate to oblong or obovate, 10 to 30 cm long, the base narrowed, sessile or short-petioled. Calyx green, 1 to 1.5 cm long, enlarged in fruit. Corolla white and pink, about 5 cm long. Capsule ovoid, 1.5 to 2 cm long.

Cultivated throughout the Philippines, in some provinces very extensively.

Dried leaves are used as styptic, sedative, emetic and purgative. The juice of the leaves is antispasmodic and a powerful insecticide. Tobacco leaves, heated, are applied to the abdomen in colic. Decoction of leaves is anthelmintic, parasiticide, for the itch and ringworm of the scalp as a local application. The leaves are used for relieving pain in rheumatic swellings and for skin diseases.

Alkaloid in leaves = 2; saponin in leaves = 1; fatty substance in leaves = 1.

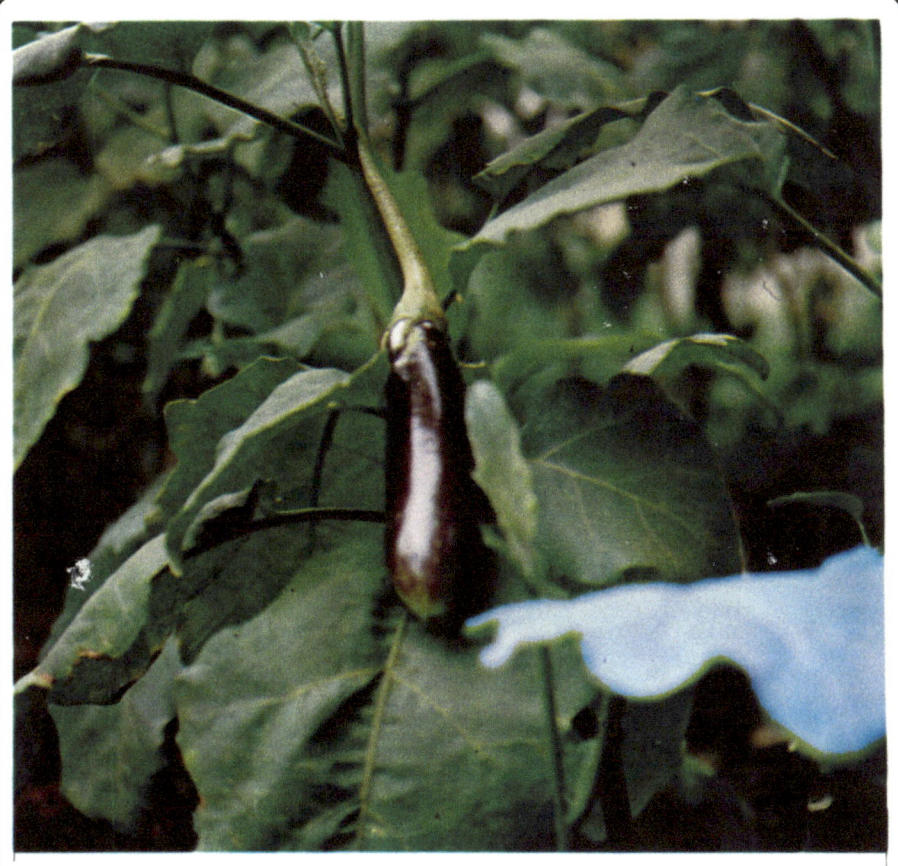

SOLANACEAE
Solanum melongena L.
Talong (Tag., Bik., Bon., Bis.); *Berengena* (Sp.); *tolung* (Sul.); *tarong* (Ilk.); eggplant (Engl.).

A coarse, usually branched, erect annual 0.4 to 1 m high, somewhat prickly or unarmed. Leaves ovate to oblong-ovate, stellate-pubescent beneath, irregularly and shallowly lobed, 10 to 25 cm long. Flowers axillary, about 2.5 cm long, purplish or bluish. Fruit fleshy, smooth, purple, up to 25 cm long, very variable in shape, globose to oblong or cylindric-oblong.

Cultivated for its edible fruit in most tropical and temperate countries.

Decoction or infusion of the leaves is a remedy for throat and stomach troubles; also used as anodyne. The leaves, roots and dried stalk are used in decoction for washing sores. Decoction of roots is taken internally as an anti-asthmatic and as a general stimulant. The fruit is antiphlegmatic, for coughs and loss of appetite; bruised with vinegar, it is used as poultice for abscesses.

Alkaloid in leaves and stem = 1; tannin in leaves = 1, stem = 2.

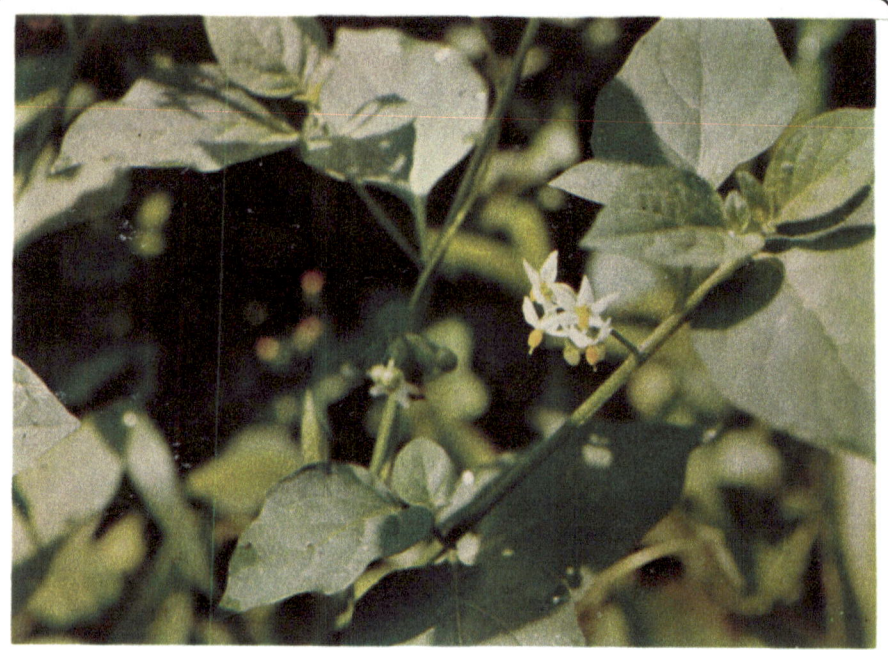

SOLANACEAE

Solanum nigrum L.

Kunti, onti, kamakamatisan, gama-gamatisan, lubi-lubi (Tag.); *bolagtab, hulabhub, lagkakum* (Bis.); *kuti* (Bik.); *amti* (Bon., If.); *anti* (Bon., Tag.); *kamatis-manok, malasili* (S.L. Bis.); *muti* (Sul., Buk.); *natang-ni-aso* (Ig.); *nateng* (Iv.); deadly nightshade, black nightshade (Engl.).

An erect, branched, glabrous or nearly glabrous herb, 1 m high or less. Stem green, somewhat three-angled. Leaves ovate to oblong, petioled 5 to 8 cm long, acuminate, base acute or acuminate, margins sub-entire or undulately lobed or toothed. Peduncles extra-axillary 1 to 2.5 cm long, the flowers umbellately disposed, five to eight on each peduncle, nodding. Calyx green, the lobes ovate-oblong. Corolla white, about 8 mm in diameter. Fruit a dark-purple or black, glabrous, globose, fleshy berry about 5 mm in diameter.

Widely distributed in the Philippines in waste places.

Infusion is used as an enema to infants with abdominal upset. A paste of the unripe berry is used as an application to ringworm. The juice or a decoction of the herb made into an ointment is used for ulcers. A poultice of the plant is applied for the relief of abdominal pain and inflammation of the urinary bladder. It is used as a condiment, stimulant, an irritant, a tonic and a febrifuge.

Alkaloid in leaves and stem = 1; glycosides in berries = 1; fats in stem = 1.

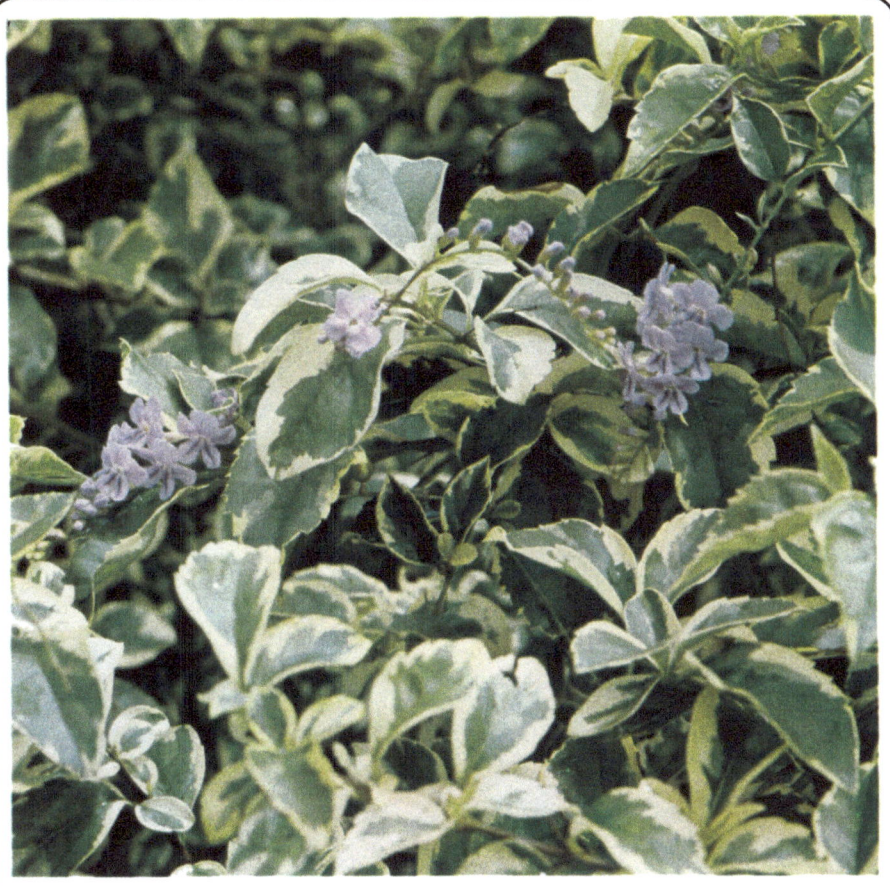

VERBENACEAE
Duranta repens L.
Duranta, golden drew drop (Engl.).

An unarmed, glabrous, erect shrub 2 to 3 m high, the branches often droop-ing. Leaves obovate-elliptic, 3 to 6 cm long, apex acute or rounded, base cuneate, margins toothed above the middle. Racemes axillary and forming terminal panicles, spreading, slender up to 12 cm long, the flowers mostly on one side of the rachis. Flowers purplish-blue, about 1 cm long, the limb about 1 cm wide. Fruit fleshy, ovoid, yellowish green, 7 to 8 mm long.

Introduced from tropical America.

The fruit is poisonous. The flowers have stimulant properties. Infusion of the leaf is diuretic, and antipyretic.

Saponin in leaf = stem and berries = 2. Sulfur in leaf, stem, berries = 1; fats in leaves and stem = 1; tannin in berries = 2; glycosides in berries and stem = 1.

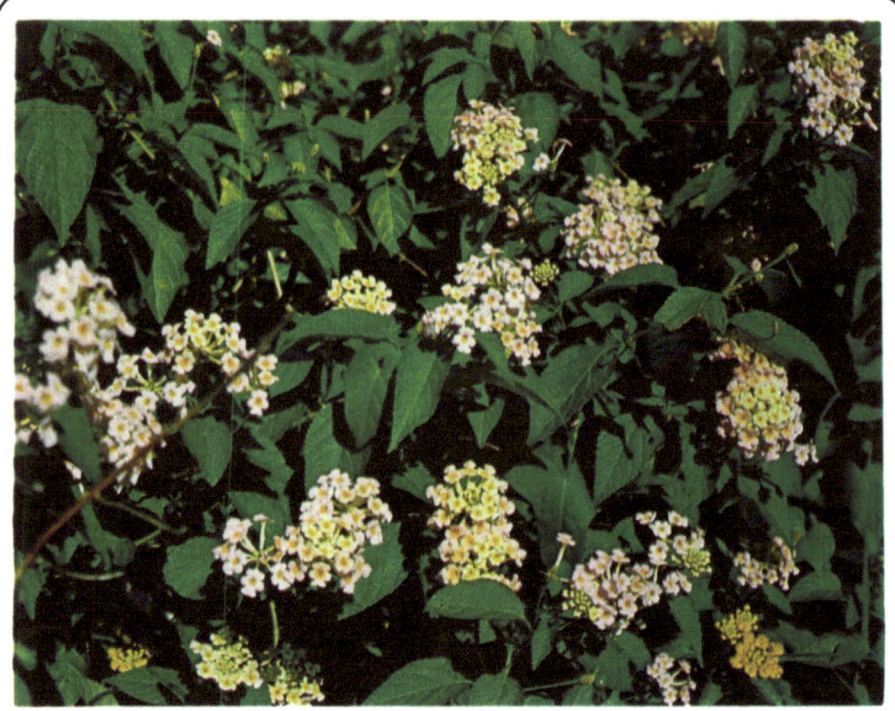

VERBENACEAE
Lantana camara L.
Lantana, sapinit, koronitas, kantutay (Tag.); *baho-baho* (Bis.);
bahug-bahug (P. Bis.); *coronitas, cineo-negritos, albahaca de caballo*
(Sp.); lantana, white sage (Engl.).

An erect or subscandent, somewhat hairy, aromatic shrub, when erect usually 1 to 2 m high, when scandent twice as high. Leaves ovate, acuminate, toothed, 5 to 9 cm long. Flowers in peduncled many-flowered heads including the corollas 2 to 3.5 cm in diameter. Corolla pink, red or yellow, about 1 cm long, the limb 6 to 7 mm wide. Fruit is an ovoid, 2 cm long, on a thickened, fleshy receptacle, purple or black, fleshy, about 5 mm long.

Abundant in waste places, thickets, etc., widely distributed and recently used as ornamental in the Philippines.

Decoction of fresh leaves and stem is used as an external wash in eczema. Pounded fresh leaves applied as poultice in sprains. Decoction or infusion of the leaves and flowering tops is used for coughs, colds and fever, a diaphoretic and stimulant; for jaundice and chest diseases; also a bath for rheumatism. Decoction of fresh roots for influenza, cough and mumps; also used as a gargle and wound wash.

Alkaloid in leaves and stem = 1; saponin in leaves = 1, stem = 2; tannin in stem = 1; fats in leaves and stem = 1-2; calcium oxalate in leaves and stem = 1.

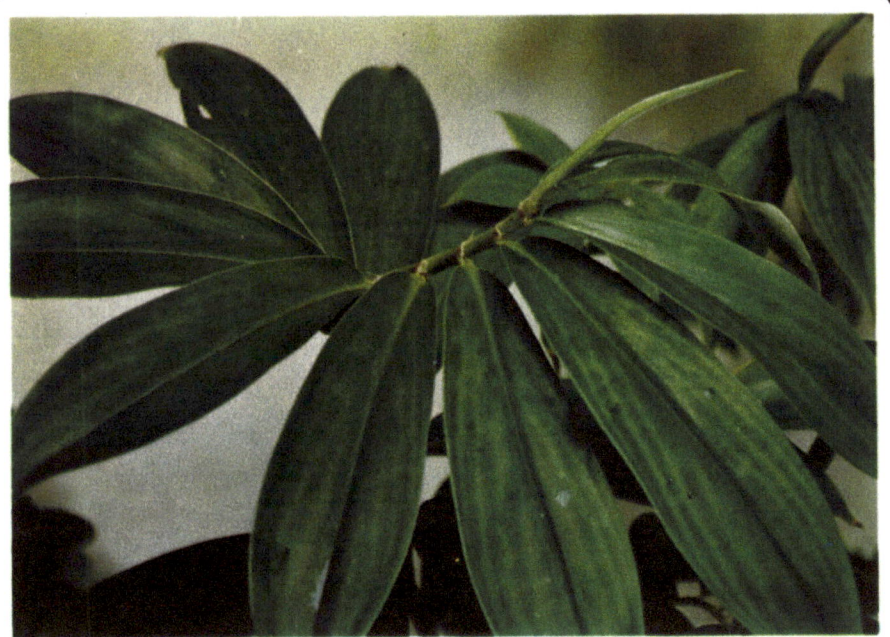

ZINGIBERACEAE
Costus speciosus (Koenig) J.E. Smith.
Tutubungiau (Bis.); *setawar* (Malay) spiral ginger (Engl.).

Stem stout, about 1 m high and 1.5 cm in diameter, leafy. Leaves spirally arranged, oblong, acuminate, subsessile, about 30 cm long, softly pubescent on the lower surface. Spikes solitary, terminal, ovoid, very dense, 5 to 8 cm long, the bracts ovate, acuminate, purple, 3 to 4.5 cm long, Calyx flattened, purple about 3 cm long, the lobes three, rather short, ovate. Corolla-segments white, oblong, 5 to 6 cm long, pointed. Lip white, sub-orbicular 6 to 8 cm long, crinkled, irregularly and rather finely toothed, the margins incurved and meeting. Stamen flat, including the broad connective about 5 cm long, 12 to 15 mm wide. Capsule ovoid to globose, red, crowned by the persistent calyx, 1.5 to 2 cm long.

Cultivated as ornamental, widely distributed in the Philippines.

The juice of the stem is given in dysentery. The roots are bitter, astringent, stimulant, digestive, anthelmintic, depurative and aphrodisiac. It is also useful in fevers, coughs, dyspepsia, worms and skin diseases. Juice of the fresh rhizome is found to be purgative. The root is used in snake-bite. The plant has antipyretic and diuretic properties.

Tannin in leaves and stem = 1, rhizome = 2; saponin, rhizome = 1; calcium oxalate in leaves and stem = 1; sulfur in leaves, stem and rhizome = 1; peroxidase in leaves, stem and rhizome = 1; amygdalin, stem = 1; amylodextrin, stem = 1; starch in leaves = 2, stem = 2-3; iron in leaves and rhizome = 1.

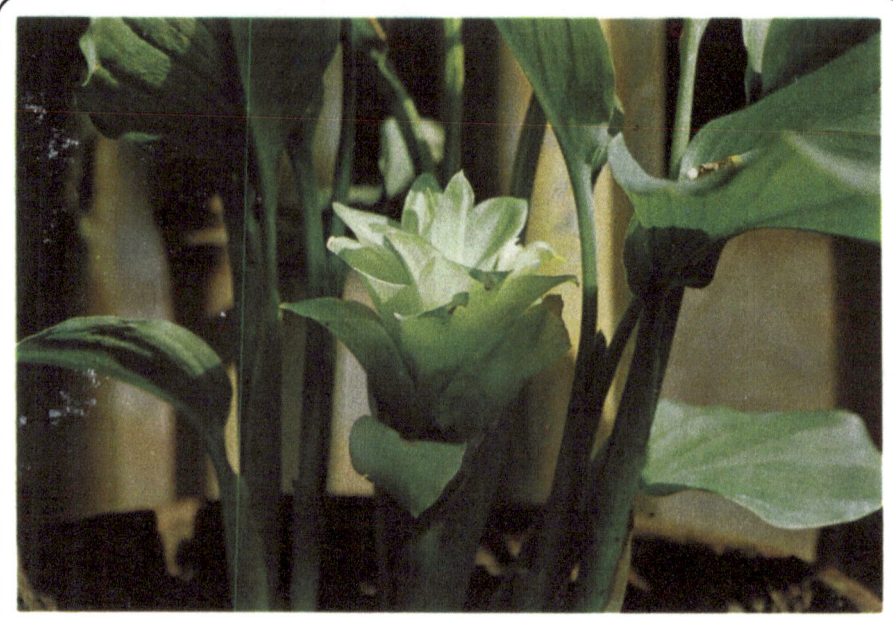

ZINGIBERACEAE
Curcuma zedoaria (Christm.) Rosc.
Barak, bolon, luya-luyahan, tamahiba, tamo-kansi (Tag.); *konik, langkauas langkuas* (Ilk.); *tamahilan* (Bik.); *tamo* (Pamp., Tag.); *koniko* (Bon.); *alimpuyas, alimpunying* (C. Bis.); *lampoyang* (P. Bis.); *ganda* (Sbl.); *unig* (If.); zedoary, zedoary root, long zedoary, turmeric, zitterwusel (Engl.).

Rootstocks stout, fleshy, slightly aromatic, pale-yellow, with oblong tuber like branches. Leaves usually in pairs, erect, petioled, green often with a purplist blotch in the center, elliptic oblong to oblong-lanceolate, slenderly acuminate, 25 to 70 cm long, 8 to 15 cm wide. Scape from the roostocks, not from the leaf tuft, often appearing before the leaves, the peduncle 10 to 20 cm long, covered with few loose bracts. Spike cylindric, 5 to 8 cm diameter, 10 to 15 cm long, composed of numerous ovate to obovate somewhat spreading, rounded bracts, the lower ones green, more or less tipped with pink, the upper ones usually longer and purple, each containing several flowers, the lower ones opening first. Calyx small. Corolla-tube 2 cm long, yellowish white sometimes tinged with purple. The tip usually yellow, two-lobed.

Found in thickets and open places; widely distributed in the settled regions of the Philippines.

Juice of the fresh rhizomes is an effective remedy in certain forms of dermatitis. Rhizome is used as gastro-intestinal stimulant in flatulent, colic and other debilities of the digestive organs. Ash of the rhizomes is applied externally to wounds, ulcers and sprains.

Alkaloid in rhizome = 1-2; calcium oxalate in leaves = 1-2, petiole = 2; glycosides in rhizome = 1; sulfur, rhizome = 1-2; fats in rhizome = 1.

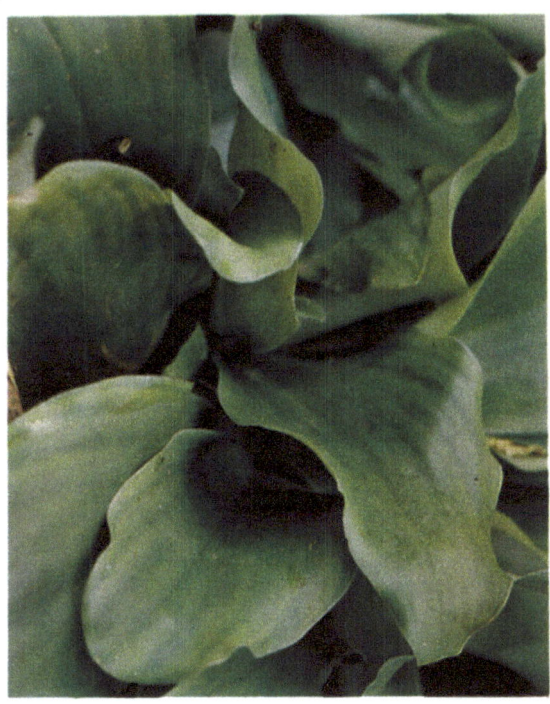

ZINGIBERACEAE
Kaempferia galanga L.
Duso, dusog, dusol, gisol, gusol (Tag.); *disol* (Ilk.);
kosol (Bis.); *kusol* (Pam.); *doso* (Bon.); *kisol* (Buk., Bis.).

A glabrous, stemless herb from tuberous aromatic rootstock. Leaves horizontally spreading, orbicular to broadly ovate, acute, obtuse or broadly acuminate, 7 to 15 cm long, base rounded. Flowers few, 4 to 6 or more, pink, the bracts lanceolate, about 3.5 cm long. Corolla-tube slender 2.5 to 3 cm long, the tip cleft to the middle, about 2.5 cm wide, white or pale pink spotted with violet. Staminodes obovate, about 1.2 cm long. Staminal-crest quadrate, two-lobed.

Widely distributed in the Philippines.

Decoction of rhizome is tonic, for dyspepsia, headache, malaria chills; applied to wounds; used in gastric complaints and carminative; also expectorant, stimulant, and diuretic. Rhizome mixed with oil is an effective cicatrizant; roasted, it is applied on rheumatic joints; rhizomes are used as a wash for dandruff or scabs on the head. Powdered rhizome is applied to wounds, bruises to reduce swellings and also to mumps and cancerous swellings. The leaves as a topical are applied externally for sore throat.

Alkaloids in leaves, root and rhizome = 1-2; tannin in roots = 1; saponin in roots = 1; calcium oxalate, leaves and rhizome = 1; iron in rhizome = 1; fats, leaves, root and rhizome = 1-2.

GLOSSARY

Abortifacient – causes abortion or miscarriage.

Accrescent – enlarging with age, as with the budscales of some flowers.

Achene – a small, dry, indehiscent one-seeded fruit in which the ovary wall is free from the seed.

Active principle – the chemical component of a crude drug which has a therapeutic effect.

Acuminate – tapering to a prolonged point.

Adnate – with unlike parts congenitally grown together.

Alkaloid – a type of complex organic compound which occurs naturally in plants.

Alternative – a substance which alters a condition by a gradual change toward restoration of health.

Amenorrhea – absence of menstruation.

Analgesic – pain-reliever or pain-killer.

Anesthetic – causes total or partial loss of sensation.

Anodyne – soothing, eases pain.

Anthelmintic – expels intestinal worms.

Antiblenorrhagic – preventing or relieving gonorrhea.

Anticolic – relieve abdominal pain by expelling gas from the stomach and intestines.

Antidote – agents which counteract or destroy the effect of poisons or other medicines.

Antidyspeptic – acts against nausea due to indigestion.

Antiherpetic – drug for skin inflammations.

Antipyretic – substance that lowers body temperature; used against fever.

Antirheumatic – medicine for rheumatism.

Antiscorbutic – used against scurvy.

Antiseptic – an agent for destroying or inhibiting pathogenic bacteria.

Antipasmodic – prevents or relieve muscular spasms or cramps.

Antitussive – an agent that relieves coughing.

Aperients – herbs which are gently laxative.

Aperitive – stimulates bowel movement; laxative

Aphrodisiac – stimulates sexual desire.

Areola – a small area marked out on a surface; a small pit.

Aromatic – emits fragrant odor; used to make medicinal preparations more palatable, also foods.

Arthritis – inflammation of a joint.

Astringent – shrinks tissues and prevents secretion of fluids from wounds.

Balsamic – healing or soothing agent.

Bitter tonic – stimulates salivary flow; used to increase appetite and aid digestion.

Bract – the small leaf or scale from the axil of which a flower or its pedicel proceeds.

Bulbs – modified plant buds which occur beneath the soil.

Cachexia – a condition of general ill health.

Calyx – outermost envelope of the flower, consisting of a number of sepals.

Capsule – a dry fruit of two or more carpels, dehiscent by valves.

Carbuncle – a deeply situated staphylococcal infection producing multiple adjacent draining skin sinuse (cavities or channels).

Carminative – expel gas from the alimentary·canal.
Carpel – unit structure of a compound pistil.
Catarrh – inflammation of nose and mucus membranes, with cough.
Cathartic – causes cleansing of the bowels.
Cholagogue – increases the flow of bile.
Cicatrizant – causes formation of scar tissue, healing of wounds.
Clavate – club-shaped, slender below and thickened upward.
Concoction – a preparation from crude materials, made by combining differ-
    ent ingredients.
Condiment – a sauce or relish for food.
Conjunctivitis – inflammation of the inner surface of the eyelid.
Contusion – injury to tissues caused by blunt force which did not disrupt or
    lacerate their surface; bruise.
Cordate – heart-shaped.
Coriaceous – leather-like; tough.
Corolla – petals of a flower.
Corymbose – a more or less flat-topped raceme in which the pedicels of the
    lower flowers are longer than those of the upper ones.
Counter-irritant – produces a blister or irritation to relieve an existing erup-
    tion elsewhere.
Crude drug – any drug, whether of vegetable or animal origin which has not
    undergone any chemical change but rather only some physical change
    such as drying and comminution.
Cupule – the cup of such fruits as the acorn; an involucre composed of bracts
    adherent by their base at least.
Cuspidate – tipped with a sharp and stiff point.
Cyme – a flat or convex, open, compound flower-cluster, the inner flowers
    opening first.
Cystitis – infection of the urinary bladder and/or urinary tract.

Debility – weakness.
Deciduous – falling off; applied to those trees that shed all their leaves at
    a particular season.
Decoctions – solutions representing the water-soluble constituents of plant
    drugs prepared by boiling the drug in water.
Decongestant – tending to reduce congestion or swelling.
Decurrent – a leaf which extends in a ridge down the twig below the point of
    insertion.
Dehiscent – a fruit that burst open upon maturity.
Demulcent – soothing medicine; provides a protective coating on membranes.
Deobstruent – clears obstructions of natural ducts of the body.
Depurative – purifying agent; normally applied to blood-purifiers.
Dermatitis – inflammation of the skin.
Detergent – cleansing agent.
Diaphoretic – induces excessive perspiration.
Dichotomous – branching by constantly forking in pairs.
Digestive – aids digestion.
Distichous – two-ranked.
Diuretic – helps the body dispose of excess water by increasing the amount
    of urine produced.
Dosage form – a preparation devised to make possible the administration of
    medication in measured or prescribed amounts.
Dropsy – edema; excessive accumulation of fluid in body tissues.
Drupe – a fleshy fruit with a hard stone.

53

Dysentery — inflammation of the large intestines with evacuation of liquid, and bloody stool and tenesmus.

Dysmenorrhea — painful menstruation.

Dyspepsia — indigestion characterized by nausea.

Dysuria — difficult discharge of urine.

Ecbolic — alleviates menstrual aches and pains.

Eczema — inflammatory skin disease characterized by redness, itching and formation of scales and crusts.

Edema — abnormal accumulation of fluids in the tissues.

Elephantiasis — disease caused by infestation with a parasitic worm; characterized by the skin's becoming hard and fissured like that of an elephant's and enlargement of the affected part of the body.

Elliptic — leaf that is oval with narrowed to rounded ends.

Embrocation — liniment of medicine for external application.

Emetic — causes vomiting.

Emeto-cathartic — causes vomiting and bowel movement.

Emmenagogue — an agent that promotes menstruation.

Emollient — softening, soothing application to the skin.

Enema — any liquid preparation introduced into the rectum.

Epiphyte — a plant growing on another plant, but not nourished by it.

Emeto-cathartic — causes vomiting and bowel movement.

Emmenagogue — an agent that promotes menstruation.

Emollient — softening, soothing application to the skin.

Enema — any liquid preparation introduced into the rectum.

Epiphyte — a plant growing on another plant, but not nourished by it.

Equitant — folded over as if astride; used for conduplicate in which the leaves are folded together lengthwise in two ranks.

Eupeptic — promotes good digestion.

Expectorant — promotes ejection of fluid from the lungs and trachea.

Exerted — protruded beyond, as stamens beyond the tube of the corolla.

Fascicle — a closed cluster or bundle of flowers, leaves, stems or roots.

Febrifuge — a remedy for fever.

Flatulence — gas formation in the alimentary canal.

Fluid extracts — liquid preparation of vegetable drug containing alcohol as a solvent or as a preservative or both.

Follicle — a many-seeded fruit derived from a single carpel, splitting longitudinally down one side.

Fomentation — application of warm, moist substances such as wet cloth to ease pain and inflammation.

Frutescent — shrubby.

Furuncle — local pus-forming inflammation of the skin and subcutaneous tissues.

Fusiform — spindle-shaped; tapering at each end.

Galactogogue — promotes secretion of milk.

Galenical preparations — any type of preparation, whether an extract of a crude drug or merely a solution of chemicals; pharmaceutical preparations obtained by macerating or percolating crude drugs with the appropriate menstruum carefully selected to extract as thoroughly as possible only the desired principles and to leave the inert and other undesirable principles of the plant undissolved.

Gastroenteritis — inflammation of the stomach and intestine characterized by pain, nausea and disease germs.

Germicide — destroys disease germs.

Gingivitis — inflammation of the gums.

Glabrous — smooth in the sense of having no hairs, bristles, or other pubescence.

Glaucous — having the surface covered with a waxy "bloom" or powdery material that rubs off.

Glume — the floral coverings of grasses.

Gout — a disease marked by painful inflammation of the joints.

Gum — viscous fluid exuded by some plants which discolors and hardens on exposure to air and light.

Hestate — with the basal lobes turned outward.

Hemorrhoid — painful swelling formed by dilatation of a vein in the anus; usually accompanied by bleeding and constipation; piles.

Herbaceous — a plant which does not develop woody tissue.

Herpes — acute skin inflammation in which clusters of small vesicles spread from one part to another.

Hirsute — with stiff or bristle hairs.

Hypnotic — induces sleep.

Imbricate — overlapping, as shingles on a roof.

Indehiscent — not opening by valves or along regular lines.

Inflorescence — the flowerhead of a plant.

Invigorant — strengthening, energy-giving agent.

Involucre — a whorl or set of bracts around a flower, or an inflorescence.

Irritant — giving rise to irritation.

Laciniate — slashed; cut into deep narrow lobes.

Lanceolate — lance-shaped.

Latex — milky juice produced by certain plants.

Laxative — encourages defecation.

Lepidote — covered with small scales.

Liniment — a solution of an irritant drug intended to be rubbed on the skin as a counter-irritant.

Loculicidal — capsules opening by splitting through the back of each cell.

Lumbago — rheumatic pain in the lumbar region (region pertaining to the loins, part between thorax and pelvis).

Macerate — cold water extract of a plant or crude drugs.

Masticatory — a substance to be chewed, but not swallowed.

—merous — part; used with numbers to denote the number of parts, as tri-merous or 3-merous, with three parts, etc.

Mucilage — gum-like material produced by some plants; has a soothing effect on inflamed parts.

Mumps — inflammation of the parotid glands.
Narcotic — a drug, which in moderate doses allays pain, reduces sensibility,
    produces sleep; in large amounts, induces stupor, coma or convulsions.
Nephritis — inflammation of the kidnesy.
Nervine — soothing to the nerves; provides nervous relaxation.
Nutrient — nourishing substance.

Oblanceolate — shaped like an inverted lance head.
Obovate — a flat inversely ovate body, the broad end upward.
Obovoid — shaped like an inverted egg.
Otitis media — inflammation of the middle ear.
Ovoid — a solid body ovate in outline.

Palliative — alleviates or eases a condition without curing it.
Pectoral — pertaining to the chest.
Peduncle — the stalk attached to the flower.
Perianth — the floral envelope of whatever form; the calyx and corolla.
Pericarp — the body of the fruit developed from the ovary and enclosing the
    seeds.
Pharmacognosy — the study of the biology, chemistry and pharmacology of
    plant drugs and spices.
Pharmacology — the study of the action of chemicals and drugs in the body.
Pharyngitis — throat inflammation.
Pinna — the primary unit of a feather-like compound leaf.
Pinnatifid — cleft in a pinnate manner.
Pistil — female element of a flower, consisting of stigma, style and ovary.
Plicate — folded on several ribs in the manner of a closed fan, occurring in
    palmately veined leaves.
Poultice — a soft usually heated preparation spread on a cloth applied to a
    sore or inflammation.
Prophylactic — preventing against disease.
Prostrate — trailing on the ground.
Puberulent — covered with fine and short or almost imperceptible hairs.
Pubescent — hairy or downy, especially with fine and soft hairs or pube-
    scence.
Pulmonary — pertaining to the lungs.
Purgative — causing evacuation from the intestines.
Pyorrhea — discharge of pus from gums.
Pyrosis — a stomach disorder characterized by burning sensation with eructa-
    tions of acid fluids.

Raceme — a simple inflorescence in which the elongated axis bears a number
    of flowers with short stems of nearly equal length.
Rachis — the axis of an inflorescence or other body.
Rank — a row, especially a vertical row.
Reactivator — restores to a state of activity.
Receptacle — generally enlarged end of flower stalk.
Refrigerant — relieving fever and thirst.
Rejuvenator — causes renewed vitality.
Repand — wavy-margined.
Restorative — aids in regaining normal vigor.
Retuse — an obtuse-apex somewhat indented.
Revulsive — diverts disease from one part of the body to another.

56

Rhizome — an underground stem.
Rubefacient — an external skin application causing redness of the skin.

Saponin — a plant glycoside which foams in water.
Scabrid — somewhat rough.
Scandent — climbing.
Scape — a peduncle rising from the ground or near it, and bearing one or more flowers.
Sedative — calms the nerves.
Sepal — a segment of calyx.
Seriate — arranged in a series of rows.
Serrulate — a finely saw-toothed.
Sessile — without a stalk of any kind.
Setaceous — bristle like.
Soporific — induces sleep.
Spathe — a bract which encloses an inflorescence.
Specific — agent or remedy that has a special effect on a particular disease.
Spike — elongated inflorescence with sessile or nearly-sessile flowers.
Stamens — the male organs of the flower.
Stimulant — increases or hastens body activity.
Stomachic — stimulates activity of the stomach.
Stomatitis — inflammation of the mouth.
Styptic — stops bleeding with an astringent.
Succulent — leaf texture which is soft and fleshy, usually thick.
Sudorific — inducing sweat; diaphoretic.
Suffrutescent — slightly shrubby or woody.
Sulcate — grooved with deep furrows.
Suppuration — pus formation.

Taeniafuge — expels tapeworm.
Tannins — a group of astringent plant constituents.
Tenesmus — the sensation of a need to evacuate the bladder or bowels without result.
Therapeutics — branch of medicine associated with the use of remedies and the treatment of diseases.
Tincture — alcoholic extract of a plant drug.
Tonic — produces healthy muscular condition and reaction.
Tortuous — twisted; full of turns and twists.
Truncate — as if cut off at the top.
Tuber — a swollen underground stem.
Turbinate — top-shaped.
Tympanitis — inflammation of the middle ear.

Ulcer — a superficial inflammation or sore of the skin or mucus membrane discharging pus.
Umbel — an umbrella-shaped inflorescence.

Vermicide — kills worms.
Vermifuge — expels worms.
Vesicant — a blistering application.
Vulnerary — used in the healing of wounds.

Whorl — three or more structures at a node, as leaves, branches or floral parts.

57

INDEX

Nicotiana tabacum	44
Plantago major	39
Solanum nigrum	46
Strychnos nux-vomica	34

Antipyretic, febrifuge

Manilkara zapota	43
Chrysanthemum indicum	14
Costus speciosus	49
Duranta repens	47
Emilia sonchifolia	15
Euphorbia neriifolia	22
Gardenia jasminoides	40
Piper nigrum	37
Pittosporum pentandrum	38
Ricinus communis	24
Solanum nigrum	46

Anti-scorbutic

Schefflera odorata	7

Antiseptic

Gardenia jasminoides	40

Antispasmodic

Acorus calamus	6
Aloe barbadensis	33
Cymbopogon citratus	25
Gardenia jasminoides	40
Nicotiana tabacum	44

Antitussive and antiasthmatic, for bronchitis

Acorus calamus	6
Aerva lanata	5
Ananas comusus	11
Barleria cristata	3
Belamcanda chinensis	29
Chrysanthemum indicum	14
Costus speciosus	49
Emilia sonchifolia	15
Euphorbia hirta	20
Euphorbia neriifolia	22
Heliotropium indicum	28
Imperata cylindrica	26
Kaempferia galanga	51
Lantana camara	48
Mallotus philippinensis	23
Piper nigrum	37
Pittosporum pentandrum	38
Plantago major	39
Rhoeo spathacea	12
Schefflera odorata	7
Solanum melongena	45
Vernonia cinerea	17

Aperient

    Manilkara zapota   43

Aphrodisiac

    Acorus calamus   6
    Aleurites moluccana   19
    Costus speciosus   49
    Strychnos nux-vomica   34

Astringent

    Adenanthera pavonina   32
    Asystasia gangetica   2
    Costus speciosus   49
    Emilia sonchifolia   36
    Ficus elastica
    Imperata cylindrica   26

For Bladder affection

    Aerva lanata   5

Cardiotonic

    Strychnos nux-vomica   34

Carminative, anti-colic, anti-flatulence

    Acorus calamus   6
    Belamcanda chinensis   29
    Bidens pilosa   13
    Calophyllum inophyllum   27
    Chrysanthemum indicum   14
    Costus speciosus   49
    Curcuma zedoaria   50
    Cymbopogon citratus   25
    Eleutherine palmifolia   30
    Kaempferia galanga   51
    Nicotiana tabacum   44
    Piper nigrum   37
    Tagetes erecta   16
    Triphasia trifolia   41

Cathartic

    Aloe barbadensis   33
    Gardenia jasminoides   40

For Diabetes

    Ipomoea aquatica   18
    Tecoma stans   10

Diaphoretic

    Cardiospermum halicacabum 42
    Cymbopogon citratus   25
    Euphorbia neriifolia   22
    Lantana camara   48

For Diarrhea, dysentery

    Manilkara zapota   43
    Acorus calamus   6

Adenanthera pavonina	32
Bidens pilosa	13
Cardiospermum halicacabum	42
Costus speciosus	49
Cymbopogon citratus	25
Emilia sonchifolia	15
Euphorbia hirta	20
Gardenia jasminoides	40
Imperata cylindrica	26
Piper nigrum	37
Plantago major	39
Rhoeo spathacea	12
Ricinus communis	24
Triphasia trifolia	41
Vernonia cinerea	17

Diuretic

Manilkara zapota	43
Ananas comosus	11
Cardiospermum halicacabum	42
Cymbopogon citratus	25
Duranta repens	42
Gardenia jasminoides	40
Imperata cylindrica	26
Kaempferia galanga	51
Plantago major	39
Tagetes erecta	16
Tecoma stans	10

For Earache

Bidens pilosa	13
Calotropis gigantea	8
Euphorbia neriifolia	22

Emetic

Acorus calamus	6
Adenanthera pavonina	32
Calotropis gigantea	8
Cardiospermum halicacabum	42
Gardenia jasminoides	40
Ipomoea aquatica	18
Nicotiana tabacum	44

Emmenagogue

Aloe barbadensis	33
Ananas comosus	11
Heliotropium indicum	28
Ricinus communis	24

For Eye diseases

Bidens pilosa	13
Calophyllum inophyllum	27
Donax cannaeformis	35
Euphorbia hirta	20
Heliotropium indicum	28

| *Nicotiana tabacum* | 44 |
| *Ricinus communis* | 24 |

For Rheumatism, gout

Acorus calamus	6
Adenanthera pavonina	32
Aleurites moluccana	19
Asystasia gangetica	2
Calophyllum inophyllum	27
Cardiospermum halicacabum	42
Chrysanthemum indicum	14
Cymbopogon citratus	25
Kaempferia galanga	51
Lantana camara	48
Orthosiphon aristatus	31
Ricinus communis	24
Tagetes erecta	16

Rubefacient

Basella alba	9
Calotropis gigantea	8
Cardiospermum halicacabum	42
Piper nigrum	37

Sedative

Chrysanthemum indicum	14
Imperata cylindrica	26
Nicotiana tabacum	44

For Skin diseases, boils and abscesses

Acorus calamus	6
Ananas comosus	11
Calotropis gigantea	8
Costus speciosus	49
Curcuma zedoaria	50
Euphorbia hirta	20
Euphorbia pulcherrima	21
Gardenia jasminoides	40
Heliotropium indicum	28
Ipomoea aquatica	18
Lantana camara	48
Mallotus philippinensis	23
Nicotiana tabacum	44
Piper nigrum	37
Plantago major	39
Ricinus communis	24
Solanum melongena	45
Solanum nigrum	46
Tagetes erecta	16
Triphasia trifolia	41
Vernonia cinerea	17

Stimulant

| *Acorus calamus* | 6 |
| *Costus speciosus* | 49 |

Duranta repens	47
Gardenia jasminoides	40
Kaempferia galanga	51
Lantana camara	48
Piper nigrum	37
Solanum melongena	45
Solanum nigrum	46

For Stomachache

Acorus calamus	6
Bidens pilosa	13
Calotropis gigantea	8
Cymbopogon citratus	25
Eleutherine palmifolia	30
Gardenia jasminoides	40
Piper nigrum	37
Ricinus communis	24
Solanum nigrum	46
Strychnos nux-vomica	34

Tonic

Acorus calamus	6
Adenanthera pavonina	32
Belamcanda chinensis	29
Chrysanthemum indicum	14
Cymbopogon citratus	25
Gardenia jasminoides	40
Imperata cylindrica	26
Kaempferia galanga	51
Piper nigrum	37
Solanum nigrum	46
Strychnos nux-vomica	34

For Toothache

Piper nigrum	37

Vulnerary

Bidens pilosa	13
Blechum pyramidatum	4
Calophyllum inophyllum	27
Curcuma zedoaria	50
Emilia sonchifolia	15
Ficus elastica	36
Heliotropium indicum	28
Imperata cylindrica	26
Kaempferia galanga	51
Lantana camara	48
Plantago major	39
Ricinus communis	24
Schefflera odorata	7
Vernonia cinerea	17

Abbreviations for the local dialects:

Bag. – Bagobo
Beng. – Benguet
Bik. – Bikol
Bis. – Bisaya
P. Bis. – Panay Bisaya
C. Bis. – Cebu Bisaya
S.L. Bis. – Samar-Leyte Bisaya
Bon. – Bontoc
Chab. – Chabacano
Engl. – English
Gad. – Gaddang
Ibn. – Ibanag
If. – Ifugao
Ilk. – Ilokano
Ig. – Igorot
Iv. – Ivatan (Batanes)
Klg. – Kalingag
Mag. – Magindanao
Mbo. – Manobo
Neg. – Negrito
Pamp. – Pampanga
Pang. – Pangasinan
Sbl. – Sambali
Sp. – Spanish
Sul. – Sulu
Tag. – Tagalog
Tagb. – Tagbanua
Yak. – Yakan

Bibliography

Brown, W.H. 1941. Useful Plants of the Philippines. Manila. Bureau of Printing.

Cardenas, J., C.E. Reyes and J.D. Doll. 1972. Tropical Weeds. Vol. 1. Bogota, Colombia.

Claus, E.P. 1956. Pharmacognosy. Lea and Febiger. Philadelphia, USA.

Co. L.L. 1977. A Manual of Some Philippine Medicinal Plants. Diliman, Quezon City.

Featherly, H.I. 1954. Taxonomic Terminology of the Higher Plants. The Iowa State College Press. Ames, Iowa, USA.

Ferguson, N.M. 1956. A textbook of Pharmacognosy. New York. Mac Millan and Co.

Githens, T.S. 1948. Drug Plants of Africa. University of Pennsylvania.

Grieve, M. 1959. A modern Herbal. New York. Hafner Publishing Company.

Hardin, J.W. and Arena, J.M. 1974. Human Poisoning from Native and Cultivated Plants. Duke Univ. Press. Durham, North Carolina.

Johansen, D.A. 1940. Plant Microtechnique. New York. John Wiley and Sons, Inc.

Lucas, R. Nature's Medicine. London. Neville. Spearman.

Lugod, G.C. and J.V. Pancho, Undated. Medicinal Plants of the College of Agriculture Arboretum and Vicinity.

Manske, R.H.F. and Holmes, H.L. 1950. The Alkaloids: Chemistry and Physiology. 14 Vols. New York Academic Press.

Merrill, E.D. 1912. A Flora of Manila. Manila Bureau of Printing.

National Science Development Board. 1978. Philippine National Formulary. Bicutan, Taguig, Metro Manila.

Newman Dorland, W.A. 1947. The American Illustrated Medical Dictionary. W.B. Saunders company. Philadelphia and London.

Quisumbing, E. 1951. Medicinal Plants of the Philippines. Manila. Bureau of Printing.

Science Education Center Work Group. 1971. Plants of the Philippines. Univ. of the Phil. Press. Quezon City.

Sulit, M.D. 1958. Medicinal Plants used by ethnic groups of the Philippines; their preparation and application. Jour. Phil. Pharm. Assoc.

Tan, Michael L. 1978. Philippine Medicinal Plants in Common Use, Their Phytochemistry and Pharmacology. Luzon Secretariat of Social Action.

Uphof, J.C. Th. 1959. Dictionary of Economic Plants. New York Hafner Publishing Company.

Valenzuela, P. JA. Concha and A.C. Santos. 1949. Constituents, Uses and Pharmacopoeia of Some Philippine Medicinal Plants. Phil Jour. of Forestry. Bureau of Printing.

Watt, John Mitchells and Breyer — Brandwijk, Maria Gerdina. 1962. The Medicinal and Poisonous Plants of Southern and Eastern Africa. E. and S. Livingstone Ltd., Edinburg and London.